CLINICAL REMARKS

CONCERNING

THE HOMŒOPATHIC TREATMENT

OF

PNEUMONIA:

96666

PRECEDED BY

A RETROSPECTIVE VIEW OF THE ALLŒOPATHIC MATERIA MEDICA, AND AN EXPLANATION OF THE HOMŒOPATHIC LAW OF CURE.

BY

J. P. TESSIER, M.D.,

PHYSICIAN TO THE HOSPITAL SAINTE-MARGUERITE IN PARIS.

TRANSLATED

BY

CHARLES J. HEMPEL, M.D.,

FELLOW AND CORRESPONDING MEMBER OF THE HOMŒOPATHIC COLLEGE OF PENNSYLVANIA; HONORARY MEMBER OF THE HAHNEMANN SOCIETY OF LONDON, &c. &c.

NEW-YORK:

WILLIAM RADDE, 322 BROADWAY.

PHILADELPHIA: RADEMACHER & SHEEK.—BOSTON: OTIS CLAPP.—MANCHESTER, ENG.: TURNER, 41 PICADILLY.

1855.

HENRY LUDWIG, Printer, 45 Vesey-st.

PREFACE.

This little work is translated from the French of Dr. Tessier, one of the most distinguished practitioners of medicine in the capital of France, and enjoying the confidence of the government as one of its accredited physicians to a public hospital of considerable importance. As a conscientious observer Tessier felt unable to withhold from homœopathy the attentive regard with which every new idea or theory that is logically put forth, should be received; and the result has been his unqualified adhesion to the homœopathic method of treatment. His experiments extended over two important series of pathological facts, *Pneumonia* and *Cholera*, which we publish in two separate volumes. The results contained in these works, will excite attention in the minds of our allœopathic brethren, and may induce many of them to imitate Tessier's noble example. They will not fail to be rewarded for their honest devotion by a confirmation of the great fact that the homœopathic treatment of Pneumonia and of Cholera, and consequently of other acute diseases is far more successful and certain than the treatment which their own School advises for such affections.

Charles J. Hempel, M.D.

New-York, *July,* 1855.

A

RETROSPECTIVE VIEW

OF THE

ALLŒOPATHIC MATERIA MEDICA,

AND

AN EXPLANATION OF THE HOMŒOPATHIC LAW OF CURE.

In giving to the public the result of some of the clinical investigations, which I had undertaken for the purpose of establishing the efficacy or the non-efficacy of the homœopathic method of treatment, I must expect to encounter various kinds of opponents.

Some will assert that I have violated the laws of professional probity by treating as a serious science that which they consider as a system of despicable jugglery and charlatanism which should be severely interdicted by the laws.

Others will pretend that I have acted without conscience towards patients who apply in our hospitals for help, by subjecting them to a method of treatment which our schools, our academies, our most eminent practitioners have repudiated and branded as an aberration of the human mind. They cannot comprehend that a public administration which owes to the poor all the solicitude that a father feels for his children, should have allowed a physician to subject the larger number of his patient to a method of treatment which excites the indignation of the most enlightened physicians.

Others again will say that medical freedom should be respected, but that it should be rendered worthy of respect by not subjecting to the crucible of experiment theories *that are evidently absurd.*

Some will say that a trial of Hahnemann's method in our public hospitals, favors the quackery of homœopathic physicians in private practice.

Others may feel disposed to assert that the value of the

homœopathic treatment has been investigated by men equally distinguished for their science and professional honor; that they have publicly condemned this method, and that, to do over again what they have done, is to cast suspicion and doubt on their intelligence.

Others, again will say that certain classes of minds require strange kinds of nourishment, as certain vitiated stomachs digest with a relish the most repulsive articles of food.

Others, finally, will maintain that by setting aside the ruling doctrines, and by repelling the wisdom of the highest authorities of the school, we fall into the most condemnable extravagances.

I have a right to believe that these objections will be raised, because they have been raised before with a violence which I need not characterize. I shall endeavor to answer all these objections and to put a stop to all such lamentations.

It will be noticed that all these objections flow from the same origin, namely from the assertion that the doctrine of Hahnemann is absurd. Indeed, if his method of treatment is not absurd, how far is professionol honor violated by applying the homœopathic treatment in a hospital? And by what reasons could, in such a case, a wise and enlightened administration be actuated in prohibiting the freedom of medical treatment, this palladium of all scientific progress? If Hahnemann's method is not absurd, the freedom of treatment is not abused by ascertaining, by means of clinical observations, the degree of usefulness and efficacy, of which this method may be possessed. If this method is not absurd, it should be tried, and examined critically; and nobody has a right to call those who exercise it in private practice quacks. How far are they quacks rather than those who do not examine the new doctrines?

If this method is not absurd, it is quite possible that the enlightened men who have tried it in practice, and have condemned it as inefficient, have been mistaken in their investigations. Is it an insult to suppose that they may have been mistaken in spite of their acknowledged science and good faith?

If the homœopathic doctrine is not absurd, it may be studied even by those who do not belong to the order of erratic minds.

And finally, if it is not absurd, the absurdity is entirely on the side of its vehement calumniators.

All the previous objections can therefore be reduced to one single affirmation, namely: *homœopathy is an absurdity*; all the rest is sheer declamation launched by vulgar minds against a species of literature which is unpleasant to them. It behooves us therefore to inquire whether or no Hahnemann's method is really absurd.

Theoretically it is indeed impossible to treat the subject in another manner. Theory cannot convey to us any higher information. Experience, or, as we now say, practice is the only standard by which the usefulness of a system can be tried. Theory and practice have their well-defined sphere of action; the former shows whether a doctrine is generally conformable to sound sense; and by means of a practical application we determine the value of a theory. This course has always been pursued in medicine; and those who condemn homœopathy as absurd without a previous examination, do so in accordance with preconceived theoretical prejudices. I shall pursue the course which has been pursued by the opponents of homœopathy, with this difference that I shall guard myself against the misguiding bias of blind passion, and shall endeavor strictly to adhere to the legitimate demands of a scientific inquiry.

Hahnemann's doctrine pretends to constitute a general reform of therapeutics; it must, therefore, furnish a new solution of all therapeutic questions. The essential points of every system of therapeutics are:

1. Scientific determination of the medicinal properties of drugs;

2. Classification of drugs;

3. The mode of observing and classifying the indications of disease;

4. The application of drugs agreeably to these indications.

(Therapeutics being the science of the indications of disease, of the application of drugs, and of the relation of drugs to disease: it evidently follows that these four points comprize the whole doctrine of therapeutics.)

1. *Scientific determination of the properties of drugs according to the method of Hahnemann.*

Experience has shown from time immemorial that only such substances as produce rapid and marked alterations in the functions after their introduction in the human organism in health, are possessed of curative virtues in disease: hence their appellation of *remedial agents.* The complex of these drugs constitutes the Materia Medica. The first condition of arriving at a knowledge of the curative virtues of drugs, is the determination of the effects which they produce in the healthy organism. How is a knowledge of these effects to be obtained?

Nature only answers when interrogated, and only answers correctly those who know how to interrogate her. In this case man has not any thing to divine, he has to learn every thing. We may apply here the words of the philosopher of Geneva: *I know that truth resides in the facts, not in my mind which observes them; and that I shall be the nearest the truth, the less I shall indulge in theories of my own.* It is observation alone that can teach us the effects of drugs in the healthy organism. But it is evident that this must be experimental observation resulting from actual trials, otherwise we should not learn much from it. Hence it is evident that trials of drugs have to be actually instituted upon healthy persons. This is one of the cardinal points in Hahnemann's doctrine, or rather its starting-point. Is this absurd? Can any thing be more lucid, more logical, more conclusive? Every sensible person will answer no: hence the starting-point is legitimate.

But it is not sufficient to institute experiments; they have to be conducted methodically, not arbitrarily. We must not content ourselves with simply observing the phenomena which make their appearance immediately after the introduction of the drug in the organism; the prover has to watch every symptom which characterises the action of the drug, the most trifling as well as the most striking; he has to observe all the changes which the drug develops in the organism, from the commencement to the termination of its action, and has to furnish us an exact picture of the drug-disease.

Is it not evident that, in order to study the pure effects of each drug, it should not be mixed up with other drugs during the trial?

This is another rule invariably followed by Hahnemann. His Materia Medica comprises therefore a complete list of the effects which the drugs he has proved, are capable of producing in healthy persons. I ask again, is there any thing absurd in this herculean labor of forty years? To me nothing seems more scientific, more methodical, more worthy of the respect of serious physicians. Who had ever undertaken and carried out such a task? It ill behooves our puny and pitiful observers to declaim against such an immense work.

2. *Classification of drugs according to Hahnemann.*

Classifications are an admirable thing, provided varieties are not mistaken for classes, but the classes are arranged in accordance with the analogies characterizing the varieties. In medicine, both in pathology and materia medica, we have always pursued a contrary route, namely: arbitrary classes were established, first, and the varieties were *nolens volens* adapted to the classes.

Drugs have been at all times divided into three classes: evacuants, alteratives and specifics. The first class, evacuants, *is again subdivided with respect to the various routes by which nature expels the heterogeneous humors, which, if retained in the system, cause the various diseases; of these subdivisions we have seven.:* *

1. Purgatives and emetics;
2. Expectorants;
3. Errhines, sneezing medicines;
4. Uterina;
5. Diuretics;

* Chomel, *Synoptical Description of the usual Plants*, Paris, 1761.

6. Diaphoretics;
7. Anti-periodicals.

The second class, alteratives, comprises the drugs *which alter in an imperceptible manner the composition of the humors*;* of these we have eleven kinds:

1. Cephalics and aromatics;
2. Ophthalmics;
3. Stomachics;
4. Hepatics, splenetics;
5. Carminatives;
6. Astringents;
7. Detergents;
8. Aperitives;
9. Emollients;
10. Anodynes;
11. Refrigerants and incrassants.

The third class, *specifics, comprises drugs which act no one knows how*;† of these we have four subdivisions:

1. Vulneraria;
2. Vermifuges;
3. Febrifuge;
4. Antiscorbutics.

Each of these subdivisions contained substances from every kingdom of nature, especially since the reform of Paracelsus. This list may show that, in our time, the classification of drugs must have become much more arbitrary for a number of physicians, without, however, having changed its basis.

Murray, in his *apparatus medicaminum*, which is the only serious work on Materia Medica that we possess, drops the traditional classification. He classes drugs agreeably to the order that was adopted in natural history; his plants, for instance, the only part of his work that he has completed, are arranged after the method of Linné.

Since Tournefort, this reform was demanded in our country by the botanic physicians. It has not prevailed, however,

* Ib.

† Hippocrates.

and the old arrangement, with the exception of some slight modifications, has been continued.*

Hahnemann has given a very severe, but just criticism of the old classification of drugs ; he shows that every drug may belong to most classes and species, and that, in each class, it is possessed of vague and uncertain properties.

In his arrangement of the drugs of the various kingdoms, Hahnemann follows the alphabetical order. This is the pure and simple negation of the traditional order. He aimed above all things at showing the natural effect of each drug.

His disciples have observed the same method, except that they adopt with Murray the natural order of classification ; they divide drugs into three classes : †

Drugs obtained from the mineral kingdom ;
" " " vegetable kingdom;
" " " animal kingdom.

This method will undoubtedly be universally adopted, if we may judge by the course of instruction which is now pursued in the Paris School of pharmacy. Guibourt, one of the most distinguished teachers of the School, has adopted this arrangement in his last edition of the *Natural History of Simple Drugs.* ‡

The alphabetical order adopted by Hahnemann is perfectly reconcilable with the natural order, which is as simple as it is wise. So far then, as Hahnemann's classification of drugs is concerned, there is nothing absurd in his method.

3. *On Hahnemann's mode of observing and classifying the therapeutic indications.*

What distinguishes the physician from the empiric, is this, that the latter treats patients without inquiring into their state, whereas the former never acts without a motive.

* Trousseau, *traité de matière médicale et de thérapeutique ;* Paris, 1847, 2 vol. in 8.

† Jahr's Pharmacopœia and Pathology, (translated by Charles J. Hempel, M. D., and for sale by W. Radde, 322 Broadway, N. Y.)

‡ *Histoire naturelle des drogues simples*, ou Cours d'histoire naturelle professé a l'Ecole de pharmacie, 4me edition, Paris, 1849—1850, 3 vol. in 8, avec figures.

According to Galenus, the therapeutic indication shows how and where art should interfere. Indeed, all the great physicians of all ages and countries, have acknowledged positive indications as their supreme rule in the selection of drugs. Whosoever deviates from them, plunges into blind routine, or into a dishonorable scepticism, dishonorable because it is without any excuse.

According to Hahnemann, the totality of the symptoms should determine the selection of the remedial agent.

This mode of selection may seem too absolute, and is besides incomplete. It omits, for instance, to take notice of the anatomical lesions which do not strike the senses; but it is not an absurd mode.

4. *On the mode of selecting a remedy according to Hahnemann.*

The selection of a remedial agent implies in the first place the acknowledgment and perception of a binding relation between the natural symptom and the medicine. This bond between the symptoms of the disease and the remedial agent has been expressed by Hahnemann in the general formula: *Similia similibus curantur*, or "like cures like." His own observations and those of others led him to establish this formula as the true therapeutic law.

Hahnemann discovered that more or less dangerous aggravations of the symptoms ensued, if his medicines were administered at the usual doses agreeably to the principle of similarity. In the place of the large doses which he employed at first, he was gradually led to administer infinitesimal doses of the appropriate remedial agents.

In all this I do not see any thing that might be termed absurd.

Hahnemann's method not being absurd, it cannot be on account of its absurdity that it has been condemned. What are the real motives of this condemnation? One motive may be the strangeness and improbability of the facts and the ideas which Hahnemann develops. These characteristics of his doctrine cannot be denied; they strike every one who, for the first time, studies Hahnemann's system.

But a rejection based upon such causes, is not legitimate· Indeed, according to the words of our poet: *le vrai peut quelquefois n'être pas vraisemblable*, truth may often seem very little truth-like. Moreover, every unknown thing at first appears strange, for the simple reason that it was unknown when it was first brought to light. This in the common fate of almost every great discovery when it is first announced. It seems strange because it was a stranger to our minds; this is the only reason.

True, strangeness and improbability have their degrees. Auscultation, for instance, is less strange than the circulation of the blood; this is less strange than microscopic entozoa, and these again are less strange than Hahnemannian attenuations. In these we pass at once from ponderable fragments to divisions which no mathematical language is capable of defining. Strangeness and improbability here seem to have reached the highest degree.

One must lose sight of all the peculiarities of the human intellect in order to be astonished at the opposition which a method for which the members of the medical profession were not all prepared, excited in their minds. Whether we appeal to natural philosophy, to chemistry, to physiology, to pathology, there does not seem to be any thing in any of these sciences to enable us to account for the action of infinitesimal doses. On the contrary, every principle in these sciences seems to oppose and conflict with the reality of this action. In this respect the most eminent as well as the most humble men in the sciences occupy the same rank; both are impressed alike; the learned are even worse off than the uninformed, for the former are perfectly aware of the immense distance that separates Hahnemann from the ruling doctrines, whereas the latter do not even suspect it.

I am therefore not astonished at the opposition which the strangeness of Hahnemann's doctrines excites at first sight. But this opposition is not any the more legitimate on that account. Indeed, the Hahnemannian doses are not without precedents in nature, and, provided we apply ourselves to the task in good earnest, we discover a multitude of facts and laws confirmatory of those which Hahnemann has established.

In physics it is an axiom that bodies can be divided without limit. Another axiom is that the molecule has all the properties of the original body.

In chemistry is it not a well known fact that combinations take place the more readily the more bodies are divided?

In physiology all the phenomena of formation refer to infinitesimal quantities. The growth of the tissue is a striking instance of this. How much does the retina or iris of a child grow in the course of a day? Twenty-five or thirty years are required for the full development of a finger. Well! let us analyse the elements of a finger, the skin, the cellular and fibrous tissue, the blood-vessels and nerves, and then let us undertake to determine the quantity of increase of these various constituents in the course of every twenty-four hours.

Chemistry does not inform us in what respect the most virulent agent differs from the most simple. Does it explain to us the nature of marsh-miasms? Does it account to us for the infinite diversity of odors which certainly constitute infinitesimal emanations? And yet these phenomena do not astonish anybody.

This shows that the facts which Hahnemann has pointed out, do not justify the opposition which has been waged against them. A first moment of surprise or hesitation may be excusable in a thoughtful mind; but an absolute rejection à priori is a proof of mental weakness and of ignorance of natural phenomena.

Another cause why the doctrines of Hahnemann have been rejected, is that their adherents are not always posted up in the science of pathology. In one sense this argument is in bad taste; I shall therefore view it in a more serious light.

It is fortunate for medicine that we have physicians of a lower rank, pathologists who do not groan under the weight of a title, who are not compromised by truth, and who can offer to genius the hospitality of their intelligence, good will, zeal and admiration, without running the risk of losing their reputation, fortune and influence. There is a gulf between the man of talent and the man of genius; but between the obscure man and the slighted genius there is a bond, it is obscurity: he is always ready to do homage to genius who does not lay claim to any himself.

In such elevated and important arts as medicine, it is well that the spirit of innovation should be opposed, enthusiasm bridled, and error walled in. The men who occupy the highest rank, are admirably adapted to opposing to the new ideas the knowledge which they had acquired: this is their mission. Opposition and contradiction are the necessary touch-stone of every truth: no truth is solidly established until it has triumphed over serious resistance. The opposition of our eminent pathologists, and the adhesion of obscure physicians are not, therefore, a sufficient reason for a purely theoretical rejection of Hahnemann's method: on the contrary, if it is to triumph, it can only do so by conquering these two orders of antagonism.

A third cause of rejection consists in the errors which Hahnemann has committed in several important particulars; but this cause is no more legitimate than any of the former; this can be shown quite easily. The vehement opponents of Hahnemann do not know them, for they have never pointed them out. They have contented themselves with assailing Hahnemann with shallow witticisms and vulgar anecdotes. Hahnemann's errors have been lucidly shown and energetically combated by his disciples. To be convinced of this, read the work of Rau's: *New Organon.* * These errors do not, therefore, constitute legitimate causes of rejection, since they are combated by Hahnemann's own disciples, and unknown to his opponents. His disciples adhere to the doctrine while combating its errors; hence these errors, not being essential to the doctrine, are no legitimate cause of a rejection *à priori.* But, for the matter of that, let any one name a book on medicine that is not filled with errors; what

* *New Organon of the specific healing art,* by Dr. J. L. Rau, translated by Charles J. Hempel, M.D., Radde, 322 Broadway, New-York.

matters it, if Hahnemann has committed errors, so long as he is right in his general principles.

If Hahnemann's doctrine is not absurd,—if the strangeness and the improbable character of his ideas,—the inferior position of his disciples,—the errors which we discover in Hahnemann's writings, do not constitute any legitimate causes of rejection: how shall we account for the vehement rage with which his doctrine has been and is being assailed by our most eminent men? I confess, I am unable to explain this fierce persecution, because I do not understand it if I am to account for it simply with reference to the doctrine itself. I should think, though, that it is rejected *à priori* simply because it is a doctrine, a theory, a systematic arrangement of ideas. The crime of this theory is to be a theory.

In the present age doctrines, theories, systems, are condemned *à priori*, become they are looked upon as the cause of all our errors in medicine. The school which prevails now-a-days in our public colleges, academies, hospitals, rejects in the most absolute manner all theories and systems. This school does not admit that medicine is a science, and it pretends to construct this science upon new observations and facts. To admit the possibility of a great truth in Hahnemann's theory, would be to give the lie to, and reject that which had been believed, affirmed and professed during a life-time. It is much easier to condemn and ridicule Hahnemann's doctrine. It do not mean to refute such errors for the present. They are sufficiently serious to deserve a special chapter, which we shall head: *on the abuse of the numerical method in medicine.* At the same time I shall state my reasons for having adopted this heading. *

So far I have confined myself to refuting objections by answering the question: Is Hahnemann's method absurd, or it is not? It seems to me that I have shown sufficiently that this method is in no respect tainted with absurdity, and that its claims to clinical experimentation cannot be denied by any one who does not mean to violate every rule of sound

* See farther on.

sense and logic. This mode of reasoning is sufficient to justify the clinical investigations that we have instituted, and their publication so far as it seemed to us necessary in order to convince prejudiced minds. It now remains for me to explain the motives which have induced me to make a beginning of such investigations in a public hospital, in spite of all the prejudices which I had to encounter, all the interests which I had to hurt, in spite of all the little storms which such a proceeding must raise against me, and which have indeed been raised. But before explaining these motives, let me say a few words of Hahnemann's errors.

Hahnemann's doctrine may be divided into two parts, his pathology and his therapeutics. Considering each by itself, it may be said that the one contains his errors, the other his truths; his pathology is wrong, his therapeutics is correct. Homœopathy is therefore a compound of fallacies and of truths.

In pathology Hahnemann was a hippocratist. Few are acquainted with hippocratism and its dangers: the great name of the father of medicine protects the vastest and the most pernicious error in medicine. It is very appropriately expressed in this familiar saying: "There are only patients, there are no diseases." This is indeed the result to which the doctrine of Hippocrates leads us in pathology, and such a result is simply destructive of all pathology, and indeed rejects and denies it. If there are no diseases, what becomes of diagnosis, of nosography, of nosology? Are they not mere chimeras?

This is not all. Hippocratism supposing all the time that disease is the reaction of the vital forces against an enemy located in the inmost depths of the organism, the mind is compelled to seek for this enemy, and is forced into the region of a fabulous etiology. A morbific agent is required to excite a reaction, for reaction does not take place without being called out by an opposing force. Hence all these imaginary causes of disease, such as alterations of the blood, or bile, mucus, black bile, acridities, saccharine or saline substances, serosities, invisible animalcules, miasms, unknown poisons; in one word, all the etiological mythology that escaped from Pandora's box. These hypotheses are the necessary results of the theory, that disease is a process of reaction, and nothing but reaction, or that disease is something identical, an essential unit in principle.

Hahnemann was not aware of the falsity of the physiological hypothesis upon which Hippocrates based the whole edifice of medicine: he adopted the traditional errors of pathology, or rather he suffered himself to be deceived by them in the same way as so many others do. Hippocratism became the source of all his errors. Hence Hahnemann's pathology cannot be criticised or rejected, without at the same time criticising or rejecting that of Hippocrates.

The rejection of all essential diseases, the psora-hypothesis, or the doctrine that the itch is the common cause of almost every chronic malady, are ideas in agreement with the hippocratic doctrine. For psora substitute black bile, or for black bile substitute psora, and the difference will be very trifling. Such are, in my judgment, the chief errors into which Hahnemann has fallen. From these general errors result the isolated errors which we meet now and then in his writings.

Let me now state the motives that prompted me to study a doctrine which is contrary to all my past notions of pathology. What is the reason that I was not deterred from such studies by this antagonism?

We want a reform in therapeutics and in materia-medica; every practitioner has been proclaiming this truth for fifty years past. There is not a student of medicine nor a practitioner of ever so little experience that has not repeated these words of Bichat: "An incoherent agglomeration of incoherent opinions, our materia medica is, of all physiological sciences, the one where the aberrations of the human mind are most strikingly depicted. What do I say? It is not a science to a methodical mind; it is a shapeless assemblage of inaccurate ideas, of observations that are frequently puerile, of illusory means of cures of formulas that are as strangely conceived as they are pompously put together. It is said that the practice of medicine is repulsive ; I go further and maintain that, in some respects, it is not the practice of a reasonable man whenever its principles are taken from most of our materia medicas."

Pinel has been praised for having denounced the practice of mixing up drugs; but these denunciations have proved so little a reform, that at the present moment, the compounding of drugs prevails more than ever. Broussais was more thorough; he proscribed at one blow the whole of the materia medica. His pupils were a little more ignorant on this account; that is all. Such means do not constitute any reform.

If therapeutics be the art of interpreting and prescribing in accordance with the morbid indications ; and if the materia medica be nothing else than the totality of the agents by means of which the therapeutic process is carried on,—it is not difficult to perceive in what manner therapeutics and the materia medica are deficient ; on the one hand, the morbid indications are arbitrary, and on the other hand, the action of drugs is imperfectly determined. Hence, a reform in medicine should aim 1, at substituting positive for all hypothetical indications; and 2, at employing remedial agents whose action has been correctly ascertained by provings upon the healthy, and whose efficacy has been established by clinical experience.

Hahnemann's labors seem to me to have realized the therapeutic reform that has been desired by all physicians. What is particularly remarkable in his labors, are his immense experimentations concerning the effects of drugs ; it is his materia medica, this masterpiece of observation, patience and unsophisticated sense. On first beholding this prodigious work, the mind becomes confused.* We are less struck by the fact that all these phenomena were observed and classed by a single man, than by the possibility of retaining them in their order in one's memory.

* We allude to Hahnemann's Materia Medica Pura and to his Chronic Diseases, 9 vols., containing the effects of upwards of a hundred drugs proved upon healthy persons. For sale at W. Radde, 322 Broadway, N.Y.

Without this gigantic work, the formula *similia similibus curantur* would have remained a trivial affirmation, such as it had been from Hippocrates to our period. But vivified by a knowledge of the pure effects of drugs, it leads to a therapeutic reform of the highest order. I will explain how.

It behooves us first to state very clearly what Hahnemann understands by *similia similibus curantur* or by *homœopathy*. We find in Hahnemann's writings several contradictory theories which impart to the homœopathic formula various meanings different from the natural sense of the words. What can the literal formula mean, if not that medicines cure morbid phenomena similar to those which the same medicines are capable of producing in a healthy person? Nothing can be clearer and simpler than this idea. It is a general therapeutic formula which established with great precision the relation of the morbid symptoms to the remedial agents. The law of similarity, thus expressed, may be either true or false, but it is lucid and precise, and presents a positive ground for discussion and for clinical and experimental verification. And lastly, so far as pathology is concerned, his formula neither denies nor affirms anything; it agrees with hippocratism just as well as with the doctrine of the essential character of diseases.

The natural or literal sense of the formula is the one that has been adopted by Hahnemann, and upon which all his labors were based. Unfortunately the illustrious reformer did not content himself with accepting the literal meaning; he undertook to give us the reason of the law which had at first appeared to him simply as a generalization of facts, and which, in order to preserve its scientific character, should never have been presented in any other light. Hahnemann plunged into physiological hypotheses concerning the inmost nature of disease, and arrived at the hippocratic conclusion that disease is a reaction of the vital force. He explained the formula *similia similibus* by substituting the artificial reaction excited by the drug in the place of the natural reaction of the vital force against the morbific agent. The symptoms of the disease indicating in their totality the vital reaction, he opposed to these symptoms, which he called disease, a similar group of symptoms produced by the drug which he termed drug-disease. Henceforth the term disease acquired an arbitrary meaning, for a group of symptoms does not constitute a disease. This led Hahnemann to a denial of the essential nature of disease; each patient became a special malady requiring a particular application of the therapeutic law. Owing to this arbitrary interpretation of the term disease, Hahnemann was enabled to proclaim without inconsistency that he had discovered the real medicine of specifics; but they were specifics with reference to patients, and not with reference to disease, since he denies their existence. Hence resulted a deplorable confusion, and legitimate occasions for attacking the homœopathic law. Indeed, if we speak of specific treatment, every body understands by it the specific treatment of some disease in all its possible forms, not the specific treatment of each patient in particular.

Hence, by changing the general formula expressing the relation of morbid symptoms to the action of remedial agents, which, as we said before, is the true meaning of the formula *similia similibus curantur*, to a general formula of specifics, Hahnemann transformed a real scientific law into an arbitrary affirmation.

But this is not all. After rejecting the doctrine of essential diseases, which he considered as something purely nominal, he admitted a certain number of acute and chronic diseases, because they were due to some miasms, thus restoring, by means of a hypothesis about acute and chronic miasms, the natural sense of the term disease in the formula *similia simi libus*. Specifics no longer referred to patients but to diseases; thus, Mercury is the specific or simile of syphilis; Sulphur is the specific or simile of the itch; Thuja is the specific or simile of sycosis; Belladonna is the specific or simile of scarlatina; Arnica is the specific or simile of traumatic affections, and so on for a certain number of other diseases. Starting from these definitions, the true meaning of the formula *similia similibus* is this: diseases are cured by drugs which produce similar diseases in healthy persons. This formula almost implies an impossibility, for no drug is capable of reproducing the phenomena of a disease in all their totality and in the same order of succession and combination, as they developed themselves in the orginal malady.

Notwithstanding these apparent inconsistencies, it is undeniable that Hahnemann has offered a general formula expressive of the relation of the pathological phenomena to the action of the drugs. This is, in my judgment, above all criticism. Moreover, the errors which we have pointed out, are chargeable to the hippocratic philosophy, whereas the truth which Hahnemann has established, belongs to him, supposing, of course, that the homœopathic law embodies a highly important general truth, as I believe it does. What matters it whether the treatment proposed by Hahnemann, is termed specific, provided it is efficacious?

As regards infinitesimal doses, what argues in their favor is the fact, that Hahnemann was led to them gradually by experience. Prescribing his remedies in conformity with the law of similarity, which requires that the natural disease should be combated by means of an artificial drug-disease that is as nearly as possible analogous to the former, he observed that the medicine as soon even as it was administered, produced a considerable aggravation of the condition of the patient; it became therefore necessary, in order to arrive at a cure, to pass through an increase of the original symptoms which was generally proportionate to the efficacy of the remedy. Every enlightened practitioner will comprehend this. What prevents him from giving Opium in headache, or Cantharides in affections of the urinary organs, for the purpose of modifying the vitality of the affected parts, if not the fear of aggravating the evil to an extent which it is not possible to determine beforehand? This was the reason why Hahnemann diminished the dose. What seems incredible *à priori*, the more he diminished the quantity of the drug, the less violent was the aggravation, and the more certain was the cure when the remedy was well chosen. What is to be said against experience, except that it ought to be confirmed by facts so numerous and so precise, that the mind feels compelled to yield to evidence? This question of doses has therefore to be determined by observation. It may be asked, however, how happens it that these medicinal aggravations are never noticed by practitioners who prescribe their medicines agreeably to the posology of Galen or Sylvius? To account for this, we have to observe two things, one general, the other special: the first is, that things which we have omitted to notice, finally cease to excite our attention; the second is, that in the Old School method of practising, only the primitive action of the drug is resorted to. In this practice the desired effect has to be produced without any delay; the cathartic has to be at once followed by alvine evacuations, the emetic by vomiting, opium by sleep, and so forth. To effect these results, it is necessary to administer a considerable dose of the drug. This is quite different in regard to the secondary symptoms produced by the drug; these secondary symptoms will be so much more marked the less the organism had been disturbed by the primitive symptoms, unless the dose had been so strong as to saturate the organism with the drug, and to cause the secondary symptoms to follow the primary. I know from experience that certain drugs if administered according to Rasori's method, induced results similar to those of infinitesimal doses, whereas the ordinary doses of the common posology remained inert. But it is useless to insist upon these points; no arguments can replace personal experience in the matter of infinitesimal doses. Upwards of five hundred trials which I have instituted with them, have convinced me of their efficacy.

It is not difficult to comprehend, that in order to apply the law of similarity, Hahnemann had to abolish the compounding of drugs. Such compound prescriptions are in the way of all certain and positive medication. To obtain this certainty, the compound ought first to be tried on the healthy organism. But no such provings have ever been instituted, and they seem indeed unnecessary, since simple drugs are amply sufficient.

Finally, an essential point in practice, is the duration of the action of drugs. This question, which is entirely new, has been opened by Hahnemann, and concluded by his numerous and indefatigable disciples.

To resume, criticise as much as one may, homœopathy is a scientific reform of therapeutics. Thanks to the labors of this great man, what has been termed rational therapeutics, has now become a system conformable to sound sense, and what Bichat declared to be unworthy of a man of reason, now constitutes a positive and regular science.

If we consider the formula *similia similibus curantur* as the general formula expressive of the relation of the symptoms to the positive effects of the drug, the homœopathic doctrine becomes a development instead of a negation of the science of medicine. Seneca was right in saying: *eril veri quod ab antiquo remotissimum*; nothing is true which is absolutely contrary to tradition. This is particularly applicable to medicine. If Hahnemann's ideas were not in harmony with the truths which have been established by succeeding generations of observers throughout a series of twenty-four centuries, these ideas would not, in my estimation, have any serious foundation; they would be of the fantastic order of the system of Asclepiades of Bithynia, capable of momentarily reducing enthusiastic imaginations, but unworthy of taking rank among the regular and positive truths which constitute the traditional basis of medicine.

Such are the reasons which have rendered it incumbent upon me to verify the truth of Hahnemann's discovery. I have done so with all the care that I am capable of. Nothing has so far prevented me, and nothing, I trust, will prevent me hereafter from fulfilling what I consider a duty. I shall not be deterred from my course by the premature condemnations which some individuals have uttered against the generous hospitality which I have accorded to Hahnemann's doctrine. I should blush to have treated it with less respect. If a theory seems radically false, we may pass on without paying any further attention to it; but when it seems pregnant with useful truths, we are bound to treat it with becoming attention; this is all I have to say in reply to my opponents.

Reconciled with the doctrine that there are essential diseases, and that there is truth in the traditions of the Old School, Hahnemann's doctrine will become more and more lucid and productive of practical good. The minds of physicians will gradually become familiar with the new system of pharmaco-dynamics, and we will wonder, in a few years, that even the most honorable men should have tried to smother an important truth.

What may appear a sophism now, will then be considered in its true light; those who, like myself, have had faith in observation, and have not sacrificed the only just and true criterium of physicians to the danger of a few personal insults and malevolent interpretations, will then have justice accorded to them. So far as the administration of the hospitals of Paris is concerned, it will redound to their honor not to have interfered in any degree with the freedom of practice in this grave business. It affords me pleasure to forestall the judgment of the future, and to express to the friends of medical freedom all the esteem with which their liberality has inspired me.

As regards those who have censured the introduction of homœopathy into our hospitals, I am convinced that some among them have done so from motives of kindness for our patients and of respect for our profession; these will be the first to acknowledge that humanity having been the gainer, the honor of the profession cannot have been tarnished by my innovation.

ON PNEUMONIA.

PNEUMONIA is a disease of frequent occurrence, acute, serious, with well-defined characteristic symptoms; it is on this account that I have selected it as the first example of an application of Hahnemann's method to the treatment of disease. No physician will dispute either the frequency or the acute nature of pneumonia; if there be a difference of opinion regarding the gravity of the disease, it is only concerning the degree of intensity which the disease exhibits. Pneumonia sometimes gets well without treatment, but nobody as yet has maintained that pneumonia, if left to itself, does not sometimes terminate in suppuration of the inflamed parenchyma. It is well known that suppuration is tantamount to death: in this case it may well be said that the exception confirms the rule. The signs by which this disease is recognized, are generally very striking, and easily distinguished; and if I admit that we might be mistaken on a first examination I make all the concessions that can be legitimately claimed. No physician can possibly mistake a case of pneumonia when he sees his patient every morning and evening, auscultates him carefully, and watches all the evolutions of the disease with the intention of determining its true character. Is the treatment of this disease as fixed and scientifically determined as the character of the disease? I think not, and this doubt imposes upon me the duty of being very cautious in my conclusions. Thus, I shall not compare the results which I have obtained with the results that have been published by other physicians; this would be premature. All that I desire to establish is, that infinitesimally small doses of drugs and administered in conformity with the similarity of their positive effects to the symptoms of the disease, exercise an evident influence upon the phenomena, the course and termination of pneumonia.—Serious minds will infer from this that they ought to study Hahnemann's method; I have no other object in view than to provoke clinical and experimental investigations on this subject. Here is the plan which I have followed:

After studying the writings of Hahnemann and his disciples, I read the records of a number of cases treated by the new method. Having understood the meaning of the formula "*similia similibus curantur*," I had to try the efficacy of infinitesimal doses. I devoted six months to this clinical verification in such acute and chronic maladies where these trials could not possibly result in the least injury to my patients. In a few days already I had obtained the most complete evidence of the efficacy of infinitesimal doses; nevertheless I continued my experiments. At the end of six months I set about investigating the merits of the new system as a complete therapeutic method, and in this new investigation, proceeded with the the strictest precision. My experimental treatment of pneumonia required the greatest precautions. It is not by any means a slight responsibility to substitute, in the treatment of an acute disease, a new method for one that enjoys the sanction of universal experience. It was therefore necessary not to expose the patients to any danger, or else to give up the new method. It seemed to me that the difficulty might be overcome with a little patience, in the following manner:

The chief therapeutic indication in pneumonia is to

bleed the patient. A sanguineous depletion, if properly applied, brings about in this disease, in most cases at least, a well-marked remission, characterized by a decrease of the fever, and a profuse perspiration with softening of the epidermis on the hands and fore-arms. Afterwards we have to remove the pulmonary hepatization which we accomplish by means of Tartar-emetic and blisters. It would not be safe to leave the remaining inflammation of the lungs to itself; the fever would return, the treatment would have to be recommenced, and the lungs would either pass into a state of suppuration or pseudo-membranous induration. In a case where a venesection had established a remission, I ventured to administer Phosphorus instead of giving Tartar-emetic which I was in the habit of doing. The patient got well without the least rise of the disease. I repeated this experiment in several other cases with the same success.

I might have attributed these results to the energetic use of antiphlogistic means at the commencement of the disease. All that I could legitimately infer from these first trials is, that I had not done any harm, if I had not done any good, afterwards I determined to diminish the number of sanguineous depletions, and not to wait for a remission before resorting to the Hahnemannean treatment, reserving to myself the right of at once returning to the ordinary treatment if an improvement should not promptly set in. In every succeeding case I diminished the number of depletions by one, two, three or four, and began to use the new remedies more nearly to the commencement of the disease. I commenced by a dose of Aconite, followed in twelve or twenty-four hours by a dose of Bryonia, after which I gave Phosphorus. The less I bled my patients the more speedily were they relieved by the small doses. At last I made up my mind not to bleed any longer, and to give the homœopathic remedies from the first. Aconite seemed to have little effect a few hours after its first exhibition; Bryonia seemed to act with great energy; Phosphorus was useful in local inflammations that threatened to pass into the stage of suppuration. The anxiety which I endured in making these first experiments, is indiscribable. In spite of my determination to bleed, if the condition of the patient should get worse; in spite of my frequent visits to these patients, it always seemed to me that some catastrophe would take place. But nothing of the kind happened. The first patients which I treated homœopathically, all got well, and some others were speedily relieved. In upwards of two years I only lost one patient. Two other patients died, but they were brought to the hospital in the last stage of suppuration. If they are recorded in my list, they can have no possible weight in deciding the therapeutic merits of the system. Since then, I have pursued the same treatment in a large number of cases of pneumonia, and my former apprehensions have gradually been removed. I do not wish to say more, and shall let the facts speak for themselves. I beg the reader to remember that in the following cases I have neither desired to furnish an exact description of pneumonia and its various characters, nor a detailed list of the symptoms of each case and the corresponding positive effects of the remedies employed. My chief aim has been to show the nature of the disease, and the method which has been pursued in treating it. Every physician is sufficiently acquainted with pneumonia to recognize it by the signs which we mention, and to appreciate the influence which the treatment had upon the disease. By revising the cases I might have perfected the record somewhat; for whatever signs may have been omitted in the record, they were never lost sight of at the bedside of the patient. I have preferred publishing these cases precisely as they were handed to me by the physicians employed in my wards. They bear a stamp of authenticity which I prefer to the embellishments of style. I have a right to say: Here is what well-informed and conscientious young physicians have seen under my eyes: they had no other interest than that of the truth; I might even say that our common interest consisted in shutting our eyes, and condemning Hahnemann's method as inefficacious and illusory; what insults, what disgust I should have saved myself! would that the persecutions might not go beyond my own person! But alas! they have already gone farther. What a courage these young gentlemen must have possessed to risk all the brilliant prospects which their future career held out to them, by assisting me in my investigations. However, I am not concerned about them; I place their zeal under the safeguard of the honor of their colleagues. All that I can personally do for them, is, to testify to them publicly my affection and my gratitude.... I may add: *Forsan et hæc olim meminisse juvabit*, one day perhaps they may be glad to think of this testimony.

The patients whose cases we are now going to report have been subjected to the following treatment:

Their beverage was water sweetened with a little sugar, from one to three quarts a day, and of a temperature to suit their taste.

They took one or two mixtures of the medicine indicated in twenty-four hours; this depended upon the intensity of the disease and its stages.

A mixture was composed of four ounces of filtered water without sugar, in which from four to six globules of the appropriate remedy were dissolved. Aconite was sometimes administered in drop doses of the sixth attenuation. All the other drugs and all attenuations above the sixth were given in globules.

A tablespoonful of such a mixture was given every two or every three hours.

An attenuation contains one-hundredth part of medicinal substance mixed with ninety-nine parts of Alcohol; if a solid, the proportion is one grain of medicinal matter to ninety-nine grains of Sugar of Milk.

Hence the 3d attenuation is equivalent to 100^3 or one-millionth of a drop of the original medicine.

The 6th to 100^6, or a unit with 12 cyphers.
" 9th to 100^9, " " " 18 "
" 12th to 100^{12}, " " " 24 "
" 18th to 100^{18}, " " " 36 "
" 24th to 100^{24}, " " " 48 "
" 30th to 100^{30}, " " " 60 "

Or:

The first attenuation $\frac{1}{100}$ drop or grain,
" third " $\frac{1}{1000000}$ drop or grain,
" sixth " $\frac{1}{1000000000000}$ drop or grain, &c.

The remedies that have been made use of most frequently, are Aconite, Bryonia, Phosphorus, Sulphur, Belladonna, Arsenicum, Iodine.

The attenuations that have been made use of are the 6th, 12th, 15th, 18th, 24th and 30th.

FIRST SERIES.

CASES TERMINATING IN RECOVERY.

CASE 1.—Influenza of 1847.—Intercurrent pneumonia.—Bronchitis previous to the invasion of pneumonia.

Joseph Croaré, 23 years old, tailor by trade, admitted on Nov. 19th, 1847, ward St. Benjamin, No. 16.

Nine or ten days ago the patient took cold. He coughed a good deal, but did not raise anything; had a fever but no headache.

Nov. 17th, while the fever had been increasing all the time, the patient was taken with a chill, which lasted an hour and was followed by a stitch in the left side, anteriorly. On the same day the sputa became yellowish, rusty. He had no sleep, but no dreams or delirium. No diarrhœa or constipation, no vomiting or nausea.

Nov. 20th, the patient was examined, had a stitch in the left antero-lateral region of the chest.

On auscultating the chest, no respiratory murmur is heard at the base of the chest. Below the shoulder-blade a very strong bellows-murmur; higher up a rasping respiration. There is bronchotomy, a slight crepitant râle in the axilla. On the opposite side, the respiratory murmur is stronger than usual; on percussion a dull sound is discovered at the base of the left lung.

Oppression of breathing, the patient coughs frequently; the sputa is copious, viscid and rusty.

The complexion is somewhat jaundiced; the malar region is flushed, the skin hot and dry. No headache; pulse 120, not hard, but soft and full.

Abdomen not painful; a diarrhœa set in to-day for the first time. The mouth and throat are not painful, but a stomatitis has developed itself, with a whitish coating on the gums and tongue; the lips were cracked.

The tongue is broad, white on the upper surface, not very much inflamed on the edges.

ANTECEDENT CONDITION.—A few days previous to being taken ill, the patient, being over-heated, had exposed himself to a cool draught. Until now he had never been very sick. He drank and ate well, had a good room, and was moderate in all his habits.

TREATMENT.—*Aconite* 15 in solution, a tablespoonful every hour.

Nov. 21.—Pulse 100. The patient feels a little better; less oppression; the murmur under the shoulder-blade is less, but stronger above. A little diarrhœa. *Aconite* 6, as above.

Nov. 22.—Pulse 100. The patient feels very weak; strong murmur at the top of the lungs; a little diarrhœa (one stool). Stomatitis worse; less jaundice. The stitch is more in front; this morning the patient has coughed a good deal, and has had some slight nausea.—*Bryonia* 30 in solution.

Nov. 23.—The pain extends over the whole chest; pulse 100, face pale, and stomatitis still continuing; four loose stools last night. Yesterday the patient committed the imprudence to rise and go to the water-closet. The murmur continues, is very loud at the apex of the lungs; on a level with the shoulder-blade a somewhat crepitant râle is heard; it is likewise heard at the base, but less distinctly.—*Bryonia* 30.

Nov. 24.—No stool; urine thick and cloudy; pulse 70; murmur less distinct at the apex; *crepitans redux;* sputa not rusty.—*Phosphorus* 30 in solution.

Nov. 25.—The murmur is only heard at the apex, and but slightly; the *crepitans redux* is distinctly heard on a level with the angle of the shoulder-blade; fever and dyspnœa have ceased; no rusty sputa, no diarrhœa.—Continue *Phosphorus*.

Nov. 26.—No more murmur at the apex.—Broth.—Continue *Phosphorus*.

Nov. 27.—The improvement continues. No fever, no murmur, no medicine.

Nov. 29.—Complete resolution.

Dec. 1.—An allowance.

Dec. 3.—The pulse down to 50.

Dec. 4.—A slight stitch in the left side; pulse 70.—*Scilla* 6 every day.

Dec. 14.—The stitch continues.—Continue *Scilla*.

Dec. 16.—Stitch continues; plaster on left side.

Dec. 21.—Feels well; the stitch is not quite gone.—Discharged.

Reflections.—This case was a very serious one. This may be inferred from the number of the pulsations, 120, from the icteric color of the face, and from the sudden supervention of the weakness.

It has been said that the pulse was not *hard*, but *soft* and *full*. At this period I again noticed the softness of the pulse which Boërhaave points out in pneumonia, an important sign, since it prevented the great Leyden physician to bleed his patients as much as they ought to have been bled. This character of the pulse in pneumonia, which is not a constant, but a very frequent symptom, is not a mere curiosity. There are authors in our day, who recommend depletions in pneumonia as long as the pulse is hard; it is difficult to follow this advice, if one knows how to feel the pulse.

The *stomatitis* is another noteworthy symptom. Concerning both this phenomenon and its explanation, Davasse has published an interesting memoir to which I refer my readers.

Aconite does not seem to have produced any other

1*

effect in this case than a diminution of the pulse from 120 to 100. I have scarcely ever seen any other effect from Aconite in pneumonia in the full stage of the disease. It is asserted that this remedy will sometimes cut short a pneumonia in the very beginning. I have never seen this result. It should be stated, however, that, in hospitals, pneumonias are scarcely ever treated from their commencement.

If we compare the action of Bryonia and Phosphorus to that of Aconite, we find that the difference in favor of the former remedies is very striking. And yet, these drugs were exhibited in the 30th attenuation, from four to six sugar-globules in a tumblerful of water, each globule of the size of a mustard-seed, impregnated with a small portion of the liquid attenuation which contained only a decillionth fraction of the original drop, or a fraction represented by the unit followed by sixty cyphers.

I trust I shall not be called upon for an explanation of these phenomena; all I can say is: read these cases with a becoming attention and earnestness of mind.

CASE 2.—*Influenza of* 1847.—*Intercurrent pneumonia.—Bronchitis previous to the invasion of pneumonia.*

Joseph Lami, 36 years old, day-laborer, admitted Dec. 1st, 1847, ward St. Benjamin, No. 35.

INCIPIENT STAGE.—On the 24th of Nov. after carrying a heavy load, and sweating a good deal, the patient exposed himself to a cool draught. Next morning he felt unwell, but not *chilly*. He coughed and raised a good deal; went to bed and kept warm; drank a good deal of cider and tried to eat; after eating, he vomited up his meal. No diarrhœa.

Nov. 26 and 27, the oppression on the chest was much worse, and the breathing more embarrassed. The sputa was neither shining nor rusty. No headache, violent fever.

Dec. 1.—Pulse 130, violent oppression and dyspnœa. Marked stomatitis; tongue red at the edges, whitish on the upper surface, but irregularly. Constipated since Nov. 28; no vomiting nor nausea.

Respiration rather stertorous; slightly crepitant rattle at the base of the right lung. Cough frequent and painful; sputa somewhat *rusty* and *tenacious.*—*Bryonia* 6 in solution, diet.

Dec. 2.—Crepitant rattle continues at the base of the right lung and in the axilla. Dyspnœa. Stomatitis worse; constipation.—*Phosphorus* 12 in solution.

Dec. 3.—Pulse 128. No headache. Jaundiced complexion. Stomatitis; dyspnœa; stertorous breathing; paroxysms of painful cough; white and frothy sputa, not rusty. No more rattle; murmur at the apex of the lungs; no vesicular murmur in the right lung; rattle and engorgement in the left lower lung.—*Bryonia* 15 in solution. The patient is somewhat delirious.

Dec. 4.—Better. Pulse 105, softer. A slight rattle at the top of the right shoulder-blade; friction-sound on the left side. Slightly delirious.—*Bryonia* in solution.

Dec. 5.—Pulse 105. Mind somewhat confused. Considerable oppression; the patient does not raise as much as he would like; no bellows'-murmur on the right side; the resolution proceeds on this side from above downwards. On the left side a slight and very fine crepitant rattle, and a slight bellows'-murmur; raises pretty easily.—*Belladonna* 6 in solution; *Sulphur* 18 in solution, alternately.

Dec. 6.—Pulse 105, resolution on the right side; on the left side bellows'-murmur on a level with the shoulder-blade.—*Bryonia* 12 in solution.

Dec. 7.—Pulse 95. Skin moist and cooler. Stomatitis. *Bryonia* 12 in solution. Takes some milk and water.

Dec. 8.—Pulse 80.—*Crepitans redux* on the left side.—*Bryonia* 12 in solution.

Dec. 10.—Pulse 70. Increase of strength; the icteric complexion continues; the appetite is good; expectoration good; full resolution.—Two soups and broth, gum-water.

Dec. 13.—Complete resolution; the patient feels well, rather weak.

Dec. 14.—Two allowances.

Dec. 21.—Continued weakness.—*China* 6 in solution.

Dec. 30.—The patient feels well, except a pain in the ear.—*Belladonna* 6 removed it.

Discharged January 2, to resume his work.

These two cases took place at the close of the epidemic influenza which prevailed in Paris in 1847. Are they to be considered as cases of influenza complicated with pneumonia, or simply as cases of catarrhal pneumonia? Owing to the existence of the epidemic, I incline to the former opinion. I do not base this opinion on the facts only, for in catarrhal pneumonia the catarrhal irritation precedes for some days the inflammation of the pulmonary parenchyma, and it likewise differs from the true pulmonary catarrh by the intensity of the febrile motions.

In these two cases the pulmonary inflammation ought therefore to be looked upon as a mere symptom, or at most as a complication of epidemic influenza. Be this as it may, inflammations of the pulmonary parenchyma being exceedingly dangerous when complicated with influenza, I have deemed it of sufficient interest to report here these two cases, where the action of the remedial agents is perfectly evident. I am inclined to doubt, at this period, that, in the second case, the indications were correctly noticed at the commencement of the disease, or in the first case, in regard to the subsequent intercostal neurosis.

It seems unnecessary to draw attention to the fact that, in this case, the pneumonia showed itself successively on the right and left side, and that the disease was a very serious one.

CASE 3.—*Pneumonia of the left lung.*

Eugene Ducerf, 28 years, wheelwright, admitted Dec. 1st, 1847, ward St. Benjamin, No. 11.

INCIPIENT STAGE.—Had a chill last Sunday evening, Nov. 28th. No catarrh or bronchitis; the chill did not last long. The patient went to bed, and had a fever all night; felt a stitch in the side during the night. Next morning the patient tried to get up, went out; he did not cough, nor raise anything; the stitch and the fever got worse, dyspnœa and oppression supervened. Had some diarrhœa.

Dec. 1.—Pulse 124, full and soft; headache, oppression, dyspnœa especially in a vertical position.

Auscultation revealed a crepitant rattle at the base of the left lung; no sputa. General color somewhat yellowish; no symptoms on percussion. Diarrhœa, considerable stomatitis; tongue coated white, with red edges; gums inflamed and covered with a whitish lining.

The patient complains of having had cold feet for some days past.—*Bryonia* 12 in solution.

Dec. 2.—Pulse 112; diarrhœa and stomatitis continue; the oppression is somewhat less. Crepitant rattle to the level of the shoulder-blade; viscid, adhering, rusty sputa.—*Bryonia* 2 in solution.

Dec. 3.—Pulse 108; diarrhœa; stomatitis and oppression less; no more crepitant rattle at the base; bellows'-murmur on a level with, and above the shoulder-blade; crepitant rattle in the axilla. The sputa continues the same, is less copious.—*Bryonia* 15 in solution.

Dec. 4.—Pulse 100, soft; patient feels very weak;

less oppression; bellows'-sound at the apex, with slight crepitant rattle.—*Bryonia* 15 in solution in the morning; *Phosphorus* 15 in the evening.

Dec. 5.—Pulse 70; expectoration good, not rusty; no bellows'-murmur, scarcely a slight rasping respiration on a level with the shoulder-blade, less oppression; stomatitis almost gone, weakness continues.—*Phosphorus* 15 in solution.

Dec. 6.—Rasping respiration at the internal angle of the shoulder-blade; pulse 70.—Continue *Phosphorus.* A little broth.

Dec. 7.—Pulse 60; the rasping breathing continues some.—*Iodine* 12 in solution.

Dec. 9.—Pulse normal; rasping respiration. Yesterday the patient had taken Phosphorus, to-day again Iodine.

Dec. 11.—Pulse perfect; good expression of countenance; good appetite; no stomatitis. Auscultation still reveals a little rasping at the internal angle of the shoulder-blade. An allowance.—*Iodine* 12 one spoonful only.

Dec. 13.—The rasping is disappearing.—*Iodine* in solution.

Dec. 14.—Complete resolution.

Dec. 15.—No medicine.

Dec. 17.—The patient complains of a little difficulty in the chest when coughing or drawing a long breath; he feels some jerking pain in the chest. Plaster on the chest in front and behind. Three allowances.

Dec. 21.—Some pains in the side.

Dec. 22.—*Hepar-sulphuris* in solution, for the stitch in the side.

Dec. 24.—Feels a little better.—Continue Hepar.

Dec. 29.—Complete recovery.—Discharged, January 3d, 1848.

This is a very simple case of pneumonia. I commenced the treatment with Bryonia in consequence of the little good which Aconite had done me in former cases. On the seventh day the pulse came down to 70. After the tenth day it was no longer noticed. At this period we had not yet sufficiently observed the decrease of the pulse under the action of Bryonia, to bestow upon this phenomenon all the attention it deserves.

CASE 4.—*Pneumonia of the right upper lobe.*

August Plet, 36 years old, worker in zinc, admitted Dec. 14th, 1847, ward St. Benjamin, No. 17.

Dec. 7.—In the evening the patient was taken with a chill. Previous to this, the patient had felt well, did not cough, but he had been hoarse for a long time previously. For six days past he had been raising a yellow, saffron-colored matter. Had had a fever since then, and had not been able to work. Had an oppression on the chest, and pain in the right side; some nausea; no vomiting, but a little diarrhœa.

Had got wet some days ago, and had kept on his wet clothes for some time.

Dec. 15.—Pulse 100, very soft; face red, bloated, yellowish. A little stomatitis. Hoarse; no diarrhœa, no vomiting, embarrassed respiration. Auscultation reveals a bellows'-sound at the apex of the right lung; no vesicular murmur in the remainder of the lungs; dulness in all the right breast, and an acute pain in this side of the chest. Sputa thick, viscid, rusty.—*Aconite* 6 in solution.

Dec. 16.—Pulse 100, very soft; jaundiced complexion; stomatitis worse; gums swollen. Bellows'-sound on a level with the right shoulder-blade and above it.—*Bryonia* 30 in solution during the day, and *Phosphorus* at night.

Dec. 17.—Pulse 75; bellows'-murmur at the top of

the chest and in the axilla.—Continue *Bryonia* and *Phosphorus*.

Dec. 18.—No fever. Less murmur; the sputa is still a little rusty; at times a little *crepitans redux*. —Continue *Bryonia* and *Phosphorus*.—Broth.

Dec. 20.—Slight murmur; very fine *crepitans redux*. Pulse 60.—Continue *Bryonia* and *Phosphorus*. Good appetite. Two soups and two broths.

Dec. 21.—Continued murmur at the top.—Iodine 12 and Phosphorus 12, alternately.

Dec. 22.—Some murmur.—Continue Iodine. An allowance.

Dec. 23 and 24.—The same treatment; two allowances.

Dec. 27.—Complete resolution.

Dec. 30.—Feels well. Three allowances. Some wine. —Discharged January 3d, 1848.

Reflections.—This case was not very serious, since the patient was able to remain eight days without any other treatment than diet and rest without the disease getting much worse. The cure was effected without much difficulty. But could it be asserted that, if left to itself, the disease would not have terminated in suppuration? If pulmonary hepatization has been allowed to run its course for a week, does it then disappear so very easily? I think not.

I will mention another series of phenomena. In this as well as in the preceding cases, we have observed a more or less general icteric tinge, a common sign of pneumonia. This sign does not belong exclusively to pneumonia; it is common to all parenchymatous inflammations. Gendrin insists above all other cotemporaneous authors upon this icteric color in pneumonia, its extreme frequency or rather its constant occurrence in this disease. This phenomenon, observed disconnectedly from the other symptoms, and badly understood, has been considered as a sign of bilious pneumonia, which is an unmeaning disease unless we understand by it an extension of the pulmonary inflammation to the liver, in cases of inflammation of the lower lobe of the right lung. This ingenious theory agrees very badly with the presence of this icteric tinge in pneumonia of the upper lobes.

CASE 5.—*Compound pneumonia.*

Louis Alfred Charron, 14 years old, admitted Dec. 14th, 1847, ward St. Benjamin, No. 13.

The patient came to the hospital for a bronchitis that had distressed him a good deal for several years past, and attacked him at intervals. No signs of phthisis.

The patient sleeps in a cold room, which is in a part of the building known as *the barracks*.

Dec. 21.—Chill, violent fever.

Dec. 22.—Sub-crepitant rattle in both sides of the chest; normal expectoration; pulse 120.—Broth, *Aconite* 6 in solution.

Dec. 23.—The rattle is finer, more towards the left; rusty sputa; pulse 120.—*Bryonia* 6 in solution.

Dec. 24.—Bellows'-sound on a level with the left shoulder-blade; pulse 110.—Continue *Bryonia.*

Dec. 25.—Bellows'-murmur and crepitation on both sides.—Continue Bryonia.—Pulse 80.

Dec. 27.—Pulse 70; bellows'-murmur on both sides, principally on the left; sputa almost normal.—*Bryonia* 15 in the day-time; *Phosphorus* 15 at night.

Dec. 29.—Pulse 70. Less murmur.—Continue *Bryonia* and *Phosphorus.*

Dec. 30.—Murmur almost gone, the boy feels smart. —*Bryonia* in solution; two broths.

During the following days perfect convalescence.

The patient remained with us as sick-nurse.

REFLECTIONS.—I will simply notice the rapid sinking of the pulse under the action of Bryonia, in spite of the intensity of the local affection which yields, itself, very speedily. Is it common to see the fever decline while the hepatization is going forward?

CASE 6.—*Pneumonia of the left lung.*

Jules Despeaux, aged 18 years, painter on china, admitted Dec. 21st, 1847.

Dec. 18.—The patient was taken with a violent chill, he could not get warm. He went to bed and perspired profusely. No stitch, but oppression, and rusty sputa. Dec. 20th the patient was bled; Dec. 21st was brought to the hospital.

Dec. 22.—Pulse 110, soft and frequent. Slight stitch in the left side since yesterday evening. The patient is strong, plethoric; face red, bloated. Stomatitis, with whitish coating; tongue white, swollen, red at the edges, with indentations. Auscultations reveals a bellows'-murmur in the whole of the left side, increasing from below upwards as far as the shoulder-blade, and most distinct above it. The cough is not frequent dyspnœa considerable. Rusty, shining, almost sanguinolent sputa.—*Aconite* 6, a tablespoonful every hour.

Dec. 23.—Pulse 90; less murmur, but continuing from below upwards; no stitch; stomatitis nearly the same.—*Bryonia* 30 in solution.

Dec. 24.—Two or three nose-bleeds. Pulse 70; tongue less swollen; stomatitis less. *Crepitans redux* below; scarcely any murmur above, more in the middle. The sputa has scarcely any color.—A little thin broth. —Continue Bryonia.

Dec. 26.—White sputa, scanty; a little murmur.—*Bryonia* in solution in the day-time, *Phosphorus* at night.

Dec. 27.—A little rasping, but neither murmur nor crepitation.—Broth and soup; Bryonia one spoonful a day.

Dec. 30.—Perfect recovery.—Two allowances.

Discharged January 3d, 1848.

In this case the patient was bled on the third day; after bleeding him, he was attacked with the stitch in the side. When he came to the hospital, the influence of the bleeding had entirely disappeared. We had to deal with a case of genuine pneumonia. The symptoms decreased as soon as we commenced to treat him, and a few days were sufficient to restore this man to his work. This is certainly not the course of a pneumonia of the whole left lung, nor is this the effect of a bleeding resorted to in the very commencement of the disease. If this bleeding had done the patient any good, he would not have caused himself to be taken to the hospital on the day after the bleeding. In my estimation the action of Aconite and Bryonia in this case is self-evident.

CASE 7.—*Pneumonia of the right side.*

Bottellier-Despoir, aged 18 years, porter, admitted January 10th, 1848, ward St. Benjamin, No. 17. His constitution was of the common order, his temperament lymphatic; had never been sick before.

January 6th, in the evening, after working hard, he stood in a draught before the door of a house to which he had taken a heavy load, and was immediately taken with a chill followed by fever and other symptoms of illness. Spent a restless and sleepless night, and next morning experienced dull pains in the right side of the chest, with labored breathing, frequent cough and blood-streaked expectoration. In this condition the patient kept his room for two days, without doing anything for himself, and not feeling any better on the tenth, he was brought to us.

Jan. 10.—Intense fever, with frequent pulse, hot and parched skin; face flushed and anxious; a slightly delirious state of mind scarcely permits him to return precise answers to our questions. Prostration of strength.

Frequent cough, with sputa of the color of the juice of prunes, viscid and copious. Breathing short and frequent. Percussion reveals a dulness in the whole extent of the posterior and right portion of the chest, and in front under the clavicle. Posteriorly no abnormal murmurs are perceived, except perhaps a rasping and puerile respiration; but in front and superiorly, from the fourth rib to the clavicle, an intense bellows'-sound both during inspiration and expiration, with crepitation at the close of an inspiration only, and during the paroxysms of cough.—Water and sugar, two pitcherfuls.

Jan. 11.—Same as before with increased dyspnœa, but no pain in the chest. Posteriorly, from the base to the apex of the lung, the bellows'-murmur had set in, with crepitation towards the base, perceptible at the close of an inspiration (bronchotomy). In front the bellows'-sound is less intense.—*Bryonia* 12 in solution.

Jan. 12.—Hurried breathing; sputa continues viscid and brownish. Pulse 124; skin dry and warm. Stethoscopic phenomena the same as before.—*Bryonia* 12 in solution.—Towards evening the pulse becomes less frequent and less strong; the skin becomes moist. About ten at night the cough begins to decrease, the dyspnœa is less distressing, the sputa, which continues viscid and bloody, is covered with a frothy serum. Pulse 96. Improvement.—Continue *Bryonia.*

Jan. 13.—Pulse 84. The sweat continues; sputa less viscid, thinner, of a lighter color. Stethoscopic signs: bellows'-murmur posteriorly at the base of the lungs, and large vesicular crepitation in the spinal depression and on its borders. In front and superiorly the bellows'-murmur has disappeared and has given place to a rasping respiration without rattle. In the evening the patient feels still better. Breathing easy, sputa full of air-vesicles and gummy.—*Bryonia* 24 in solution.

Jan. 14.—Pulse 68. Temperature of the skin almost natural; sputa still whiter and lighter. Slight diminution of the bellows'-sound posteriorly; the *crepitans redux* is heard on a level with the spine of the shoulder-blade.—Water and sugar, two broths.

Jan. 15.—Same symptoms, same treatment.

Jan. 16.—Restless night, cough worse. Sputa more copious than the day before, but mucous and opaque, floating in a quantity of serum. Sibilant rhonchus in the whole left lung, and mucous rattle in the right.—*Sulphur* 30 in solution.

Jan. 17.—The bronchitis continues.—Water and sugar, two broths, *Sulphur* as before. No fever.

Jan. 18.—No fever. Frequent cough with mucous sputa, which has the same appearance as on the previous days, but is less copious.—Water and sugar.

Jan. 19.—Bronchitis improved; mucous rattle in the right lung less.—*Aconite* in solution.

Jan. 20.—Convalescence continues very strikingly.—Two broths, two soups.

Jan. 20—29.—A little cough, mucous expectoration, but not much.—*Ipecac.* in solution. An allowance.

February 1.—The bronchitis has ceased. Discharged Feb. 7.

This case of pneumonia was at first light, but continued to get worse until the patient came under our treatment, which commenced six days after he had been taken sick. On the evening of the 12th of January a remission of the symptoms began to manifect itself, and the resolution of the local and general phenomena went on with marked rapidity. On the fourth day of the treatment, the pulse had come down to 68; the patient was able to take a little broth.

January 16th a severe bronchitis broke out; bronchitis frequently sets in after pneumonia. Sometimes this is simply a continuation of the bronchial inflammation which accompanies the inflammation of the pulmonary parenchyma; sometimes this complication is owing to some indiscretion on the part of the patient who leaves his bed for some cause, gets cold, steps with his bare feet on the floor, &c.

CASE 8.—*Pneumonia of the left side.*

Freillard, 53 years old, day-laborer, of a robust constitution and a bilious-sanguine temperament; has always enjoyed good health.

January 17th was suddenly taken with a chill, without any assignable cause, with acute pains in the loins; the chill lasted two hours, and was followed by a violent fever, cough, bloody sputa, and a painful stitch in the side, during the cough, in the left axilla. Was a whole week without treatment, had applied for admission in some hospital day after day, and could not obtain leave until this evening.

Jan. 24.—Moderate heat of the skin; pulse large, soft, from 80 to 84 beats; face bloated; intense headache; tongue coated white, with red edges; intense thirst. Respiration frequent, quick, arrested every now and then, and painful when drawing a long breath, on a level of and below the left axilla. Cough frequent, easy, followed by viscid, rusty and tenacious sputa. Percussion yields a good sound in the right side of the chest, and all over in front; on the left side, posteriorly, the sound is dull. No respiratory murmur in the superior and posterior two-thirds of the left lung, and a moist, large, vesicular rhonchus is heard towards the close of an inspiration in the corresponding inferior third; bronchophony in the same regions, more marked in the axilla than elsewhere. Puerile respiration in front.—*Aconite* in solution in the evening.

Jan. 25.—Face bloated, headache, tongue coated white and red along the borders; skin hot and dry; pulse full, from 80 to 84. Prostration of strength; no sleep;

respiration small, frequent, stitch in the side more acute than the day before; the patient has to lie on the left side, any other position being painful.

Cough loose, with copious rusty sputa, not very tenacious, and a copious greenish, frothy serum floating on top of it in the chamber.

Dulness of percussion posteriorly, and, in the same region, bronchophony, and very loud bellows'-murmur from the base of the lung to the spine of the shoulder-blade. At the latter point, and in the sub-spinous depression, a fine and copious crepitation is heard at the close of an inspiration. At the base of the lung the bellows'-sound is intermingled with a large vesicular mucous rattle which is particularly distinct during a paroxysm of cough. From time to time, on a level with the spine of the shoulder-blade, a rasping, dry noise is heard, like the rustling of silk, whence Dr. Bazin who is present at the examination, infers the existence of local and partial pleurisy. Water and sugar, two pitchers full; *Aconite* 6 in solution, and *Bryonia* 18 in solution, alternately.

Evening: same symptoms, prostration increased.

Jan. 26.—No sleep in the night, cough more frequent than in the day-time.

Headache and facial congestion less. Pulse large, soft, 80; intense thirst; temperature of the skin like that of the breath.

Breathing frequent but equal; expectoration the same. The stitch in the axilla is less painful.

Bellows'-sound and bronchophony the same; the mucous rhonchus, which was at first limited to the base of the lung, reaches the middle third; crepitant rattle less dry in the sub-spinal depression.—Water and sugar; *Bryonia* 18 and *Phosphorus* 30 in solution, alternately.

Evening; moist skin. Breathing fuller and less frequent, the serum which floats over the rusty sputa, becomes whitish.

Jan. 27.—Little headache; pulse large, compressible, 76. Profuse sweat all night, the patient had to be changed twice. Tongue coated white; scarcely any thirst.

Breathing easy, but continues painful in the axilla during a deep inspiration. Raises easily; cough not frequent, followed by copious expectoration, slightly rusty, spreading and floating in a quantity of serum.

Bellows'-sound and bronchophony posteriorly as before; mucous rhonchus inferiorly, scattering; crepitation less dry superiorly.—Continue *Bryonia* and *Phosphorus.*

Jan. 28.—No headache; feels well; slept four hours the night before; skin naturally warm. Pulse 64.

Breathing easy; the painful stitch during the cough continues; he coughs seldom and raises a yellowish substance, which spreads and floats in a quantity of serum.

A slight bellows'-sound posteriorly; no bronchophony. *Crepitans redux* at the base of the lung, along the inner border of the shoulder-blade and superiorly. Mucous rattle in the sub-spinal depression, and exteriorly.—Continue *Bryonia* and *Phosphorus.*

Jan. 29.—No fever. Pulse 60 to 64.

Breathing natural; the painful stitch continues. Expectorates a puriform mucus which is covered by a quantity of thin and white serum.

Dulness of sound less. *Crepitans redux* behind; abundant mucous rattle during the cough.—*Sulphur* 18 in solution.

Jan. 30.—Same as yesterday; less crepitation.—*Sulphur* in solution, two broths.

Jan. 31.—Same. Expectoration the same. Crepitation has ceased, in the place of which a mucous rattle is heard; little or no dulness of sound.—Two broths.

Feb. 1.—Same. The bronchial respiration reappears in the sub-spinal depression; copious expectoration.—*Sulphur* in solution, diet.

Feb. 2.—The bellows'-sound continues, and the mucous rattle posteriorly. Mucous expectoration, with frothy serum.—Continue *Sulphur*.

Feb. 3.—Yellowish expectoration in small quantity; a good deal of serum; the bellows'-sound above the spine of the shoulder-blade continues; but it has lost of its roughness.—Two broths and soups.

Feb. 6.—The bellows'-sound is almost entirely gone. Serous expectoration.—*Sulphur* in solution, an allowance.

Gradual disappearance of the bellows'-sound and expectoration. Discharged Feb. 28.

The patient in this case was not a young man of eighteen, but a stout man of fifty-three years old, who had been affected with pneumonia for eight days without having anything done for him. In his case the frequency of the pulse, 84, was not at all proportionate to the intensity of the other symptoms; the expectoration is easy and copious. The mucous rattle, intermingled with the bellows'-noise and the bronchophony, gave rise to apprehensions of suppuration, in these parts. What rendered this case peculiarly dangerous, was the absence of all treatment for the first eight days.

Two days after his admission in the hospital the improvement commenced; on the twelfth day of his disease, it was broken; on the thirteenth the fever ceased entirely.

The complete resolution of the parenchymatous hepatization did not take place at once, and the bronchial inflammation continued for some days; could this have been otherwise? At the age of fifty-three, resolutions take place slowly, especially if the disease had been progressing for a week without any treatment.

I am firmly of opinion that, without treatment, the patient would have died of suppuration.

CASE 9.—*Chronic affection of the heart.—Pneumonia of the left lung.*

Daublet, cap-maker, admitted January 24th, 1848, ward St. Benjamin, No. 26, aged 59 years, of pretty good constitution, but weakened by toil and poverty; had never been very sick until January, 1846, when he was attacked with dyspnœa and palpitation of the heart, which compelled him to abstain from work. Was never treated consistently for this affection. Having grown worse in the last fortnight, he applied to the hospital for aid. On the day when he was admitted, he had no fever, but complained of dyspnœa, palpitation of the heart and pains in the præcordial region. Striking intermissions of the pulse every third or fourth beat; it is hard and resisting. Dulness in the præcordial region over an extensive surface; considerable impulse of the heart between the fifth and sixth ribs; dull sounds heard at a distance. During the first sound, a loud and harsh bellows'-murmur.—(Gum-water and sugar, two pitcherfuls.)

During the night he was suddenly taken with diarrhœa, and went out of the hall to the water-closet; he felt cold, and in the morning, a few moments previous to my visit, he was seized with a violent chill, with a painful stitch behind and on the left side. Percussion and auscultation do not as yet reveal anything. About ten o'clock, reaction takes place; a violent cough sets in, at first dry, afterwards accompanied by a browish expectoration floating in clear serum.

Jan. 25, Evening.—Expression of anxiety and depression of spirits in the countenance. The stitch in the side is more painful, the breathing more hurried;

cough frequent, with easy expectoration of rusty sputa in little quantity, and always floating in a large quantity of serum. The whole body had a livid-yellow color. The sclerotica especially exhibits this tinge. The pulse is not so tense as it was in the morning; it counts from 112 to 116 beats; the intermissions have ceased entirely. Dulness of percussion behind and on the left side, in the sub-spinal depression; fine crepitations, especially at the base of the lung.—*Aconite* and *Bryonia* in solution alternately.

Jan. 26.—Scarcely any pain in the thorax, even when coughing. Intense dyspnœa; cough and expectoration the same as before. Icterus more striking. Skin continues dry and parched; pulse large, less resisting, 104; tongue coated white; thirst moderate. Dulness of percussion more extensive and more striking than yesterday. A good deal of crepitation on a level with the spine of the shoulder-blade, and in the axilla of the same side; sub-crepitant rhonchus below, on a level with the base of the lung; bronchial respiration along the internal border of the shoulder-blade.—*Bryonia* and *Phosphorus* 12 in solution.

Evening, 6 o'clock.—Same state. Cough less frequent, and the patient feels more comfortable; pulse large and soft, from 90 to 94. Slight moisture on the skin.

Jan. 27.—The patient slept two or three hours in the night, and had to be changed twice. No pain in the chest. Breathing easy; cough less frequent, but with saffron-colored sputa that was less copious than previously; and with less serum. Skin moist, with icteric, livid tinge; the sclerotica seems to look clearer. Pulse large, 90, with a few intermissions. Dulness of percussion, and bellows'-sound posteriorly, in the region where the crepitant rhonchus was heard.—*Bryonia* in solution.

Evening. The patient feels still more comfortable. The icterus is decreasing.

Jan. 28.—Cough rare, with viscous, saffron-colored expectoration, almost without serum. Breathing continues easy; warmth of the skin natural; the icterus has disappeared. Pulse 80; the intermissions become more marked again. Dulness of percussions behind; *crepitans redux* at the close of an inspiration, only in the axilla, and from the spine of the scapula to the base of the lung; no bellows'-sound in this region, which is only perceived, though slightly, along the internal border of the scapula.—Continue *Bryonia.*

Jan. 29.—Cough rare, with scanty, mucous sputa. Pulse 80, intermittent; icterus almost gone. Only a little vesicular crepitation here and there, without any bellows'-sound behind. The patient desires to eat.—Two broths.

Jan. 30.—Perfect convalescence.—Two broths; two soups.—The same until

Feb. 1.—An allowance. The patient remained in the room until Feb. 7, without dyspnœa or palpitation, although the signs of his organic affection remained the same as when he was first admitted.

Every body knows that a pneumonia which sets in during the existence of an organic affection of the heart, is a very serious disease. I had every reason to be forcibly impressed with the ease and quickness with which this patient was cured of his disease. I will not dwell upon the interesting signs which characterized the organic affection in this case, nor upon the changes of the pulse during and after the pneumonia.

CASE 10.—*Pneumonia of the left side.—Metastasis to the brain.*

Violat, porter, was admitted Jan. 29th, 1848, ward Saint Cécile, No. 7. This was his first sickness. He was tall, strong, of a bilious-nervous temperament; aged 40 years.

The day previous to his admission, he woke in the morning with a violent fever, not preceded by a chill, and characterized by thirst, headache, heat all over, and loss of strength; he had to remain in bed. Desirous of resuming his work in the middle of the day, he went out and was attacked with a violent chill in the street, with pain in the inferior and left posterior region of the thorax; a few turns of cough and expectoration of blood-streaked sputa. After his return home, the fever increased, the cough and expectoration became worse, especially at night; he did not sleep any. On the third day of his sickness he was admitted to the hospital.

Evening.—Violent headache, burning thirst, tongue red and dry; skin hot and parched; pulse strong, full, from 108 to 112 beats.

Breathing frequent, unequal, interrupted at times by a violent pain in the left chest, opposite the nipple.

Cough not frequent; the patient tries to suppress it in consequence of the pain; the patient raises with difficulty a little rusty sputa, which is tenacious and strongly adheres to the bottom of the vessel.

Percussion shows dulness of sound over a space of four fingers' breadth below the left clavicle, and behind in the super and sub-spinous depression; puerile respiration on the right side; a good deal of crepitation in the region corresponding to the dulness, intermingled in front, below the clavicle with slight, vesicular crepitation at the close of a deep inspiration. Bronchophony trifling.—*Aconite* 18, two tumblerfuls.

Jan. 30.—Same as yesterday, except a striking diminution of the pain in the chest; the bellows'-sound is heard only during an expiration on a level with the internal and superior border of the left shoulder-blade.

The patient raises a little rusty sputa.—*Bryonia*, two tumblerfuls.

Evening.—Flushed face, the eyes shine and sparkle, he answers hastily, and is restless.

Jan. 31.—Restless night, with slight delirium. The pulse which was full and strong the day before, has become small, hurried, jerking, from 120 to 124; skin continues dry and parched; tongue coated white in the middle and moist. Face animated, eyes staring and sparkling; his answers are short, incoherent, or he does not return any answers at all. At times the patient hides his head under the clothes, and says he is well. Pupils contracted; cough rare. Rusty sputa, in very small quantity, viscid, and raised during the night.

Slight dulness of sound in the upper portion of the chest, in front and behind.

Fine crepitation below the clavicle. No bronchophony or bellows'-sound behind, when the breathing seems natural, but feeble.—*Bryonia*, two tumblerfuls; *Belladonna* in solution, for the evening; cold ablution.

Evening.—No cough, no expectoration, no abnormal signs of respiration.

February 1.—Same condition. Delirium, fever with complete suppression of every symptom of pulmonary inflammation. Cold showering morning and night.

Feb. 2.—Same condition.—Ablution morning and night; a potion mixed with one-fourth part of Moschus.

Feb. 3.—The delirium is no longer constant; the patient has spent a few hours in the night without restlessness or crisis.

The heat of the skin is less. Pulse less rapid and larger, 100; slight moisture on the hands and in the face; the right pupil is more contracted than the left. —Cold showering. *Belladonna* 6 in solution, during the night.

Feb. 4.—No more restlessness or delirium; profuse

sweat at night and in the morning; pulse large, rather soft, 76; natural expression of countenance; dilatation of the pupils; slowness of ideas.

Evening.—The improvement continues. Pulse down to 68; skin has a natural temperature. No sweat; mind perfectly clear. The patient desires to eat.—*Belladonna* 18, in solution.

Feb. 5.—Improvement still more marked. Pulse continues to fall, down to 56.—Two broths.

Feb. 6.—Same condition.—Two broths; two soups.

Feb. 7 and 8.—An allowance. Perfect convalescence. Discharged Feb. 26.

In this case the rapid resolution of the pulmonary inflammation seems to be owing principally to the cerebral metastasis. I have controlled this meningitis by Moschus in five grain doses and cold showering; the Belladonna did not seem to reach this condition. I resumed Belladonna as soon as the symptoms indicated it distinctly, and it acted very promptly.

The combination of methods in this case shows that it is more important as regards the nosography of disease than as an illustration of the method of Hahnemann.

CASE 11.—*Pneumonia of the left lung, at the commencement of acute phthisis.*

Surbled, stone cutter, aged 61 years, of middling constitution, was admitted Jan. 29, 1848, ward Sainte-Cécile, No. 14.

At the age of 40 he had pneumonia of the right lung, and was treated at the Pitié, with venesections and Tartar-emetic, and was discharged cured after a treatment of two months. Since then his health has been good.

On the 18th of January last, he was taken with a slight chill on rising, and a feeling of weariness all over, which obliged him to keep his bed for two days. January 21st, feeling pretty smart, he went to his work; but he had scarcely commenced it when he was taken with a violent chill, followed by heat, vertigo and general weariness. His comrades gave him wine with sugar, made him drink a few glasses of brandy, and led him home. On his way home he was taken with a dry cough and a stitch in the side. He went to bed, dieted, wetted a couple of shirts, but did not feel any better. On the days following, the fever and cough grew worse; January 24th, the patient had a blood-streaked mucus. They gave him hot elder-tea to drink, and kept him in a constant sweat by covering him with an enormous quantity of blankets. But the patient continued to grow worse, and he entered the hospital January 29th.

His face was red, head heavy. He complained of stitches striking from the left to the right supra-orbital region, as far as the ears. Tongue coated white, moist; thirst moderate; mouth bitter; skin dry and burning. Pulse 104. A dull pain on a level with the left nipple aggravates the breathing; frequent and distressing cough, with a serous, vesicular expectoration, in the centre of which one perceives a small quantity of the characteristic reddish-brown sputa.

On percussing the left lower and posterior region of the chest, one meets a complete dulness of sound. In the same region, auscultation reveals a good deal of sub-crepitant rhonchus, and higher up, towards the spine of the shoulder-blade, a very harsh bronchial murmur during an expiration, and less harsh during an inspiration. Bronchophony.—*Aconite* 6 in solution; two pitcherfuls of water and sugar.

Jan. 30.—Scarcely any headache; tongue coated white and moist; temperature of the skin like that of the breath. Pulse large, dicrotus, 100 to 104.

The stitch is less; the breathing less painful; cough frequent; the rusty sputa floats in a smaller quantity of loosely coherent serum.

The stethoscopic and physical signs are the same as yesterday.

Bryonia and *Phosphorus* in solution, the former in the day-time, the latter during the night.

Jan. 31.—Bad night. More fever and cough. The heat, thirst and cough have proved very troublesome; scarcely any serum in the spittoon; only rusty sputa, mixed with a little saffron-colored expectoration; what he raises, is very tenacious.

In the morning the skin is still dry and burning, no headache, tongue coated white and moist; pulse large, soft, down to 84. No stitch in the side, the breathing is easy.

The dulness of sound behind has spread more upwards. In front, below the nipple, where the sound had remained normal so far, it has become dull. *Crepitans redux*, dry, frequent, striking the ear in large masses at the base of the lung. Bronchophony in the super and sub-spinous depressions, intermingled with subcrepitant rattle, which is only heard during an inspiration. Every now and then rhonchus is heard in these regions. The bronchophony is continual.—*Bryonia* and *Phosphorus* in alternation.

Evening.—Restless and slightly delirious; the skin is not abnormally hot, but is covered with a clammy sweat. Pulse small, quick, vibratory; tongue dry; prostration of strength. The expectoration becomes very copious. The sputa is less tenacious and rusty.—Sinapisms on the calves.

Feb. 1.—Has been restless and delirious all night. Gummy expectoration which fills one-third of the spittoon.

Copious sweat at six o'clock in the morning; the patient has been changed three times.

During the forenoon the skin remains covered with sweat; tongue coated white and moist. Pulse large, undulating, down to 76. Crepitation in the whole posterior portion of the lung.—*Phosphorus* in solution.

Feb. 2.—Skin moist; pulse 64, soft; feels comfortable.

Profuse mucous expectoration.

Crepitans redux less frequent than the day previous. A normal respiration is beginning to be heard at the base of the lung. The bellows'-murmur on a level with the internal and superior angle of the shoulder-blade continues.—Two broths.

Feb. 3.—Same symptoms.

Feb. 4.—Same symptoms. Bronchial murmur in the same region; mucous expectoration.

Feb. 5.—Same symptoms.—*Sulphur* 18; two broths.

Feb. 6, 7, 8, 9.—Bronchial murmur and copious mucous expectoration.—*Sulphur* and *Ipecac.* in alternation. An allowance.

Feb. 14.—The murmur has become harsh, and is intermingled with a little vesicular crepitation here and there. Cough more frequent, especially in the evening. The sputa becomes thicker; the dulness of sound has completely disappeared below, and continues above. In the night the patient feels oppressed.—*Hepar-sulphuris* 18 in solution.

Feb. 15 to 17.—These symptoms are growing worse. Every evening a little rise of fever, not preceded by a chill, but followed by night sweat.

Feb. 18 to 26.—Fever every evening, loss of appetite; emaciation; mucous sputa, homogeneous, floating on top of a clear liquid. Dyspnœa increasing.

Complete dulness of sound, and cavernous rattle in the specified region. The phenomena of phthisis are becoming more and more apparent. The hectic fever, the night sweats, the expectoration, and finally the diarrhœa, hasten the dissolution of the patient, who died of marasmus on the 19th of May, 1848.

Post-mortem examination.—Strong adhesions between the costal and pulmonary pleura behind and in front. The lower lobe of this lung is engorged, and has the color of claret-sediment. The upper lobe contains in its centre a vast tuberculous cavity filled with a greyish fetid matter, and having sinuous borders. The surrounding tissue presents a general infiltration of tuberculous matter.

This case is peculiarly interesting as regards the pneumonia and the phthisis, and their mutual relation.

The pneumonia had been allowed to run on, or nearly so, until the ninth day. For two days the treatment was accompanied by a slight improvement; on the third day of the treatment a crisis sat in; the pneumonia was broken. The fever disappeared and a general resolution took place, except in one point, where new symptoms show themselves, after the convalescence had continued for a fortnight. These new symptoms were the signs of an acute phthisis that took the patient off at the end of three months and some days.

An acute phthisis after a pneumonia is not unfrequent in old people. I have met it in some cases at the Hotel Dieu, but always among men. I have never seen it among old women, even at the Salpetrière, although I had a good many cases of pneumonia in that institution. This may only be an accident. This is not the place to discuss this form of phthisis.

CASE 12.—*Pneumonia of the left lung.*

Koch, a teacher, 67 years old, of middling constitution, had been for some time in the ward St. Benjamin, No. 2.

Feb. 6.—Koch was taken in the night with an intense fever, without any precursory symptoms, and without any assignable cause. Slight headache, flushed face, intense thirst, red tongue, hot and dry skin, pulse 112; frequent respiration; slight oppression and a dull difficulty of breathing in the left side of the thorax. No cough, no expectoration, no stitches. Dulness of sound below the left shoulder-blade; striking diminution of the respiratory murmur, in the same region, but without their character being at all altered.—*Aconite* 6 in solution, diet.

Feb. 7.—The fever is the same; the pulse is softer.

Respiration frequent and small; oppression worse. The dilatation of the thorax during an inspiration is scarcely perceptible on the left side, although it takes place without any local pain

Cough rare, dry.

Dulness of sound from the spine of the left shoulder-blade to the base of the lung.

Complete absence of all respiratory murmur in the two lower thirds of this region. In the upper third a tubular bellow's-murmur is beginning to be heard towards the close of an expiration.

No rattle either dry or moist.—*Aconite* 6 in solution.

Feb. 8.—Sleepless night; tongue moist and covered with a whitish coating; red edges. Intense thirst. Pulse large, soft, less frequent (about 100). Skin dry and warm.

Respiration small, incomplete, but painless; the sick portion of the chest is scarcely moved.

Cough rare, with expectoration on several occasions, of a little saffron-colored viscid sputa strongly adhering to the bottom of the vessel.

The dulness is more perceptible than the day previous.

At the base of the lung, behind and interiorly, towards the close of an inspiration, the crepitating sound of a few fine vesicles is heard; and, on a level with, and on the inner side of the sub-spinous depression the tubular bellows'-murmur and bronchophony are very striking.—Continue *Aconite;* water and sugar.

Evening.—The skin is not so dry, the patient expectorates with difficulty a little rusty sputa.—*Bryonia* 18 in solution.

Feb. 9.—Less thirst; tongue coated white and moist; skin moderately warm; pulse soft, 84.

Breathing fuller and slower.

Cough increased, but not frequent, with viscid, not very copious sputa, some rusty, some saffron-colored.

Dulness behind.

Bronchial respiration in the whole posterior portion of the chest. Imperfect bronchophony at the base, very striking on a level with the spine of the scapula.

Complete absence of rattle.—*Bryonia* 18, two solutions.

Feb. 10.—No thirst; tongue coated white; warmth of the skin almost natural; pulse soft, 80.

Breathing slow.

Cough rare, with viscid, saffron-colored sputa, mingled with more copious thick mucous sputa.

Dulness continues.

The tubular bellows'-murmur is less harsh, intermingled at the close of a deep inspiration with a mucous rattle at the base of the lung, and a fine, abundant crepitation above.—Continue *Bryonia*.

Feb. 11.—Fever ceases entirely; temperature of the skin natural; pulse 72.

Respiration normal.

Cough more frequent in the night, with expectoration of a considerable quantity of thick sputa. *Crepitans redux* in the two upper thirds of the affected lung; an abundant mucous rattle in the lower third. Bronchophony ceases.—Continue *Bryonia*.

Feb. 12.—Continued improvement. Cough and expectoration the same.—Water and sugar, two pitcherfuls.

Feb. 13.—Return of fever; the patient had gone out

of the room to the water-closet. Thirst, red tongue, heat of the skin; pulse 80, resisting.

Cough not frequent, moist; profuse expectoration of mucus. The dulness behind continues.

Harsh respiration, and large vesicular mucous rattle in the sub-spinal fossa at the base of the lung. Puerile respiration under the clavicle of the same side.—*Bryonia* in solution; water and sugar.

Feb. 14.—Profuse sweat at night. In the morning the skin is moist, pulse large, expectoration less copious and partly serous.

Respiration continues harsh, also the mucous rattle behind.—*Bryonia* and *Phosphorus* in solution, alternately. Broth.

Feb. 15.—Sweat all night until this morning. Cough and expectoration less. Diarrhœa over night.—Broth.

Feb. 16.—No fever. Cough and expectoration have almost ceased; very little mucous rattle; diarrhœa continues.—*Rheum.* in solution; diet.

Feb. 17.—Two stools over night, the patient had again left his bed; cough worse, with more mucous expectoration; abundant mucous rattle; reappearance of bronchophony on a level with, and on the inside of the spine of the left scapula.—*Phosphorus* in solution; diet.

Feb. 18.—Rise of fever last evening; copious sweat at night. Less expectoration.

Dulness continues, with mucous rattle and bronchophony. Water and sugar; diet.

Feb. 19.—No fever. Skin and pulse natural, 60; diarrhœa reappears; the patient raises a little vesicular mucus; no bronchophony; fine and circumscribed *crepitans redux* in the sub-spinal depression.—*Rheum.*; water and sugar.

Feb. 20.—Diarrhœa less. Scarcely any cough or expectoration; crepitation at the close of an inspiration, only in the region indicated; harsh respiratory murmurs any where else.—Continue the same treatment; two broths.

Feb. 21.—Gradual convalescence. Cough and diarrhœa cease. Feb. 24.—Has an allowance; still a little dulness and harsh respiration, but decreasing every day.

In the beginning of March he had a fall on the left trochanter major, which caused a considerable swelling of the upper portion of the thigh, with inability to move this limb (an intra-capsular fracture). At the end of March the swelling had disappeared, and the motion of the limb ceased to be painful. But the limb remained so weak that the patient was unable to stand upon it; he kept his bed and remained in the hospital for months after, enjoying otherwise perfect health.

In this case, as in many other cases, Aconite does not seem to have proved efficacious. An improvement set in after the first dose of Bryonia.

The complete resolution of the hepatization was delayed by the indiscretions committed by this patient. This poor fellow who was very timid, and was kept in the ward on account of his poverty, dared not apply to the nurses when he had to satisfy a call of nature, and went into an icy cold corridor to the water-closet, in spite of all our entreaties to the contrary.

CASE 13.—*Pneumonia of the right side.*

Nereu, day-laborer, 47 years old, was admitted Feb. 7th, 1848, in the ward St. Cécilie, No. 11. This patient had a robust constitution, and had never been sick.

On the 4th of Feb. on going to bed, he felt ill, and was taken with alternate chills and flushes of heat which continued all night. In the morning, the fever had fully set in, (with anorexia, thirst, headache, heat all over,) and was soon followed by a dry, distressing cough, with a dull sense of embarrassment rather than any real pain in the right side of the chest. Next morning, these symptoms were still worse, and the cough is followed by expectoration of a blood-streaked sputa. The patient was bled, and then came to the hospital.

Feb. 7.—Violent fever. Headache, flushed face, dry tongue and skin, with intense thirst; pulse 120, quick, tense; slight trembling of the extremities.

Painful stitch in the side on a level with the edge of the false ribs of the right side, aggravated by the cough, which is frequent, short, with bloody sputa which is surrounded with a clear serum and is difficult to raise. Breathing painful.

Dulness of sound behind over the two lower thirds of the right side, and in the axilla. Intense bellows'-murmur in the same region, and crepitant rattle at the base of the lung which becomes particularly frequent during a deep inspiration. Marked bronchophony.—*Aconite* 18, two tumblers full; water and sugar, two pitcherfuls.

Feb. 8.—Same as yesterday; the patient had a restless night, and distressing dreams when the momentary cessation of the cough allowed him a short nap.

Skin less hot, pulse less tense, fuller and less frequent, 100.

Sputa more copious, less red, more viscid and rusty, with a large quantity of serum floating above it.—*Bryonia* 24, two tumblerfuls.

About four o'clock in the afternoon, the skin becomes slightly moist. The headache and cough are less.

Feb. 9.—Had a bad night; restless, slightly delirious; fatiguing cough.

Morning visit.—The skin is very hot and dry, pulse large, compressible, 90; tongue dry and red; little or no headache. The stitch is painful only during the cough; this is less frequent, shorter, with profuse expectoration of viscid rusty sputa, without serum. Dulness the same in quality and extent as on the previous days. Bronchial respiration continues harsh and labored. The crepitation at the base of the lung seems to rise towards the upper portion, and to extend over a larger surface. It is heard both during an inspiration and expiration. In the right axilla the crepitation is very fine and abundant.—*Bryonia*, two solutions.

In the evening, increase of fever; intense thirst and headache. Pulse hard, tense, quick, about 100; dyspnœa. Respiration hurried, panting; cough dry, hoarse; no expectoration since this paroxysm commenced, which was about two o'clock. About nine o'clock in the evening, the exacerbation of the previous symptoms decreases, the expectoration recommences; a slight moisture breaks out on the face and hands.—Sinapisms on the legs.

Feb. 10.—Spent a better night. Tongue coated white and moist; no headache; skin very warm but not excessively dry; pulse large, undulating, compressible, 84.

No stitch in the side; respiration normal; cough easy, profuse expectoration of gummy sputa; the tubular murmur and bronchophony are limited to the super and sub-spinous depression. Fine *Crepitans redux* in the remaining portion of the inflamed lung.—*Bryonia* and *Phosphorus* in solution, alternately.

In the evening, the patient had three diarrhœic stools, and filled the chamber half full with a red urine depositing a sediment. The skin is moist all over, without being exactly sweaty.

Feb. 11.—Had a quiet night, the patient says he feels perfectly comfortable. Tongue coated white and moist; warmth of the skin mild and pleasant. Pulse large, depressible, 80 to 84. Cough rare, easy; profuse mucous expectoration; general *crepitans redux*, with bronchial respiration without harshness all along, and especially above the outer border of the scapula.—*Bryonia* in solution.

Feb. 12.—Skin natural, pulse 60. Mucous sputa.—*Bryonia* two spoonfuls a day.

Feb. 13.—Perfect convalescence. Crepitans redux perceptible only at the close of an inspiration. Slight bellows'-murmur above. Mucous expectoration less.

Feb. 14.—Same condition.—Continue *Bryonia*; two broths.

Until Feb. 20th the bellows'-murmur is heard in the sub-spinal depression, and the patient takes a solution of *Phosphorus* every other day. Gradually resumes his customary regime. Feb. 22, perfect recovery. Two allowances; discharged March 4th.

This was a serious case of pneumonia. It terminated in a discharge of critical urine on the seventh day, after very alarming signs. The bleeding to which the patient was subjected to in the commencement, had no effect. The sinapisms which were applied on the evening of the sixth day, are an important circumstance. By facilitating the diaphoresis and preventing a metastasis to the brain, they contributed a good deal to the successful termination of the disease.

During the course of this disease, Bryonia was never given below the 24th attenuation. This was probably too high. Nevertheless its action seems to me evident. Under its influence, the pulse came down at once twenty beats; on the ninth day it was down to 60, after having been 120 on the fourth day. At this period we were not yet in the habit of noting the successive decrease of the number of beats after the resolution had set in. In the following cases the effects of Bryonia in this respect will be pointed out more fully.

CASE 14.—Cortial, porter, aged 39 years; ward St. Benjamin, No. 8.

Had a good constitution, a sanguine temperament; is

not subject to any hereditary diseases, and has never been seriously ill heretofore.

In the evening of the 10th of February, after working hard, he was taken with wandering chills mingled with flushes of heat, weariness and restlessness. This continued all night. In the morning had a fever, intense headache, thirst, without any other characteristic symptom. Spent the whole day and night in this state, without taking anything but water and sugar, until the afternoon of the second day, when he was taken with a dry and fatiguing cough, and causing a constantly increasing, acute pain on a level with the lower angle of the right scapula. Gradually the cough became moist, and was followed by yellow, viscid, blood-streaked sputa. No treatment.

Feb. 15, evening, was admitted to the hospital. Violent fever, flushed face, tongue moist and coated white; thirst moderate; skin dry and burning, except in the palms of the hands, which are very moist; pulse strong, full, 100. Prostration of strength, he is scarcely able to give an account of his anterior condition.

Dyspnœa; respiratory movements unequal, irregular.

Cough not frequent, painful.

Difficult expectoration of bloody sputa, not very tenacious and floating in an equal quantity of a whitish loosely coherent serum.

Percussed in front, the right side of the thorax yields a normal sound, behind, from above downwards, and in the corresponding axilla, percussion yields a striking dulness. A moderate percussion of the chest excites a pain towards the base of the lung.

Auscultation reveals harsh tubular respiration, especially during the expiration, with bronchophony from the lower angle of the scapula to the sub-spinal depression, being particularly striking along the internal border of this bone, and gradually decreasing in going to the armpit, where a crepitating rattle is heard.—*Aconite* 12 in solution, two tumblers full.

Feb. 16.—Fever the same as last night, except the thirst, which had become more intense; the face was less flushed and bloated; less headache. Pulse 104, large and full.

Dyspnœa not altered; respiration continues unequal, and is more painful behind than on previous days. The patient is better able to lie on the right side. Cough more frequent, difficult and painful.

Expectoration more copious, sputa less red but more tenacious. Part of the sputa is rusty; it is all mixed up with a quantity of frothy serum which floats on top.

Stethoscopic signs not changed.—*Bryonia* 18 two tumblerfuls. Water and sugar.

In the evening, violent rise of fever. Pulse quicker, small, tense; dyspnœa with occasional interruption of breathing. The patient is extremely anxious and restless; the tubular murmur is scarcely heard in the region where it was heard yesterday morning, probably on account of the deficient dilatation of the affected side of the thorax which is almost immoveable. Cough and sputa are scarcely changed any.

Between 10 and 11 o'clock in the evening, the anxiety, oppression and fever are less; the pulse is slower and quieter; the cough is less painful, the expectoration looser and more copious.

Feb. 17.—This improvement continued during the night. Next morning the patient exhibited the following condition:

Scarcely any headache; tongue coated white and moist; thirst moderate; pulse quick, but not resisting, 100; warmth of the skin mild; a little moisture on the forehead.

No more dyspnœa. The respiration is quick but neither irregular nor intermittent.

Stitch in the side continues painful at the close of an inspiration, and during the paroxysms of cough.

Cough very frequent and painful.

Easy and copious expectoration of viscid, rusty sputa, surrounded by a serous liquid as previously.

Marked dulness at the posterior portion of the chest, and in the axilla of the same side. Percussion has ceased to be painful.

Bellows'-murmur and bronchophony very distinct in the same region and over the same surface.—Continue *Bryonia;* water and sugar.

In the evening, the patient feels better. The stitch is scarcely any longer painful; sweat had commenced to break out at two in the afternoon, and at this moment it has become general, but not copious; pulse large, soft, compressible.

Feb. 18.—Spent a good night; the patient had to put on a dry shirt. No headache in the morning; tongue moist and coated white; thirst moderate. Skin soft, moist; pulse large, undulating, 90. The patient feels well; no oppression; respiratory movements regular and natural.

Stitch has almost ceased.

Cough easy, not very frequent; copious expectoration of saffron-colored sputa, not so tenacious, and mixed up with a quantity of serum.

Dulness continues.

The tubular murmur and the bronchophony have developed themselves under the right clavicle; behind they are not very distinct, and the *crepitans redux* is heard here during the cough and at the close of an inspiration.—*Bryonia* and *Phosphorus* 18 in solution, alternately.

Feb. 19.—Skin soft and moist; since last night the patient had to be changed twice. Pulse soft, 90; tongue moist and white-coated.

Respiration normal; stitch not very painful, and only when coughing.

Copious sputa, either saffron-colored and viscid, or mucous and opaque, with a little serum.

Dulness behind, not very distinct in front, under the clavicle; bellows'-murmur in this region; abundant crepitation in the whole posterior region.—Continue *Bryonia* and *Phosphorus*.

Feb. 20.—No sweat; temperature of the skin natural; pulse 80 to 84.

Cough frequent, easy, expectoration the same, except no serum, and decrease of the saffron-colored sputa.

Dulness in the same region.

Crepitans redux in front, not very striking behind, where the normal respiratory murmur is heard on a level with the sub-spinal depression.

Feels quite comfortable. The patient desires to eat. —*Sulphur* 18 in solution.

Feb. 21.—Copious mucous expectoration; mucous rattle at the top of the lungs in front; respiration feeble behind, and mucous rattle at the close of an inspiration.—Continue *Sulphur*.

Feb. 22.—Less expectoration; the sputa is of a lighter color, and partially vesicular; pulse 70 to 72.—Continue *Sulphur*. Broth.

Feb. 23.—The expectoration continues to diminish.

Feb. 24.—Perfect convalescence.—An allowance.—Discharged March 6th.

A case of true pneumonia; no treatment until the sixth day. Aconite is given; not much improvement on the morning of the seventh day. *Bryonia* is followed by an aggravation in the afternoon; in the evening a remission of the symptoms set in, which continues to the end. Phosphorus is given alternately with Bryonia to hasten the resolution of the pulmonary hepatization. On the sixth day of the treatment, the patient feels quite well. Is not this testimony sufficient?

CASE 15.—*Pneumonia of the right side.*

Baudot, 48 years old, day-laborer, of a robust constitution, and a sanguine temperament; admitted March 20th, 1848, in the ward Sainte-Cécilie, No. 11.

Has had a cold for a fortnight past; coughs a good deal at night, in the morning raises a little phlegm. No fever, but had to keep his room for a few days. The bronchitis having got better after this period of rest, he returns to his work.

On the 19th of March, while going to Alfort with some of his companions, he perspired on the way, and took cold after his arrival. He was suddenly seized with a violent chill, followed by fever, a dry and violent cough, and an acute pain on a level with the right nipple. In the night these symptoms got worse, and the oppression and the cough became so violent that the patient was afraid he might suffocate.

March 20, on coming to the hospital, bloated face, dull headache, slight icteric color of the sclerotica. The tongue is red, dry; thirst intense. Skin burning hot, pulse hard, tense, 116 to 120; anxiety; cough dry, frequent and painful. The patient tries to suppress the paroxysms in order to avoid the aggravation of the stitch in the side. The breathing is rapid, short, sometimes interrupted and irregular; the oppression very striking.

Percussion yields an obscure dulness on a level with the two lower and posterior thirds of the right lung. In this same space there is a complete absence of the respiratory murmur, and a slight diffuse bronchophony. In front, on the same side, the respiration is feeble, but on the opposite left side it is puerile.—*Aconite* two solutions; water and sugar two pitchers full.

Feb. 21.—Restless night. Cough less distressing,

with a little red, viscid sputa, strongly adhering to the vessel.

In the morning, the fever is intense; dull headache, the face no longer bloated; a general icteric color has developed itself.

Tongue red, skin burning and dry; pulse 116; prostration of strength; the patient is scarcely able to set up.

Marked oppression; rapid, unequal respiration; the right side of the chest almost remains unmoved. Cough frequent, painful, with occasional expectoration of bloody and very tenacious sputa. Stitch in the side continues painful.

Behind, on a level with the lower angle of the scapula a slight bellows'-murmur is heard; the bronchophony is more distinct; during the cough, or at the close of a deep inspiration, a crepitant rattle is heard scattered over a surface.—*Bryonia* 18 two solutions, two pitcherfuls of water and sugar.

In the evening, the cough becomes more and more moist; the sputa is of a lighter color, and more copious. The bellows'-murmur is very distinct on a level with the lower third of the lung; and quite low down crepitant rattle is heard.

Febr. 22.—The night has been pretty good.

Icteric color. The headache is much less. Tongue coated white and moist; warmth of the skin like that of the respiration; pulse large, strong, less frequent (100).

Breathing easier; the respiratory movements are regular and uniform; but the right side does not dilate. The stitch in the side remains the same.

Cough frequent and followed by easy expectoration of copious, tenacious, rusty sputa.

Tubular respiration from the spine of the scapula to

the base of the lung, along the internal border of the bone. Sub-crepitant rattle low down.

Evening: moist skin. The patient feels better; discharges a large quantity of sedimentous urine.

Feb. 23.—Sweat in the night; copious discharge of sedimentous urine.

In the morning, the tongue is coated white and moist; no headache. Icterus ceases; only the sclerotica remains yellow. Pulse large, soft, down to 80 or 84.

Breathing easy; stitch in the side scarcely perceptible. Cough less frequent; scanty saffron-colored sputa.

Same dulness and over the same surface as on the first day. The bellows'-murmur is only heard on a level with, and interiorly to the spine of the scapula. Below, a fine and abundant *crepitans redux*. Bryonia, three spoonfuls a day, water and sugar.

Feb. 24.—The icterus has disappeared. Pulse soft, compressible, 72.

Cough rare; mucous expectoration not very abundant.

Bellows'-murmur and crepitation the same as yesterday.—Continue *Bryonia.*

Feb. 25.—Bellows'-murmur less. Crepitation scattered; tongue coated white; heat of the skin natural; pulse 72.

The patient desires to eat.—Two broths.

Feb. 27.—Bellows'-murmur scarcely perceptible.—Respiration at the base of the lung normal.—Two broths, two soups.

Perfect convalescence on the following days. The patient remains for some weeks in the ward as a laborer, and leaves it May 2d.

The remarks appended to the last case, equally apply to this one. The exhibition of Bryonia was followed by an immediate and continual improvement without aggravation.

CASE 16.—*Pneumonia of the right lung.*

Calson, aged 33 years, locksmith, of ordinary constitution and nervous temperament; admitted in the ward Sainte-Cécile, No. 13, April 18th.

Had been subject to epileptic attacks since his boyhood; first they consisted in a little momentary nervous derangement, but, for the last ten years, having increased to characteristic paroxysms, setting in without precursory symptoms, at irregular periods and long intervals. These paroxysms had not as yet affected his intellectual or organic functions, and, except his disease, Colson had always enjoyed good health.

Was attacked with small-pox at the age of 18 years.

Last week, at a period which he did not exactly recollect, he was taken with a sick feeling, loss of appetite, weariness in the extremities. Continued his work nevertheless.

On the 4th of April, in the afternoon, this indisposition assumed a serious character. Without any assignable cause, he experienced a difficulty of breathing, with a few paroxysms of dry and distressing cough. In the evening he had chills followed by heat, vertigo and general soreness and weariness.

On the following days he kept his bed, with a hot fever, an acute pain opposite the right nipple, and a distressing cough followed by bloody expectoration. He had not had any treatment.

Calson came to the hospital on the fifth day of his sickness; he showed the following symptoms:

Pale face, sparkling eyes; staring look; sudden, but correct and precise answers; dry tongue, covered with a dry and yellowish coating in the middle, with red edges; bitter taste; occasional nausea; not much thirst.

Skin warm but soft; moisture on the forehead and in the palms of the hands. Pulse large, full, 112 to 116.

Dull pain on a level with the right false ribs, worse

when coughing. Respiration easy, but frequent; expectorates a small quantity of viscid, saffron-colored, opaque sputa.

Marked dulness under the right clavicle and decreasing gradually as far as on a level with the fourth rib, where it ceases; behind, in the sub-spinal fossa, it is only heard in consequence of the resonance from the opposite side.

In the same space is heard the tubular murmur with a few crepitating vesicles around the nipple and in the axilla; behind none of these abnormal murmurs are heard, even during a deep inspiration.—*Aconite* in solution.

April 9.—Restless and delirious all night.

In the morning, the face looks animated; his eyes stare, his answers are short and sudden; he gets angry at being taken for a sick person; he is constantly repeating that he is getting better, and he raises himself suddenly to have his chest explored.

Tongue a little moister, scarcely any thirst.

Pulse 112. Skin warm. The patient does not complain of any pain in the side.

Cough rare; a little viscid sputa, of a yellow-brown color.

Same physical signs.—*Bryonia* 12, two solutions.

The delirium continues in the day-time; the patient uncovers himself constantly, and the force-jacket had to be put on him. In the evening his face is covered with sweat, likewise the lower extremities which are the only ones that can be examined. During the night the delirium decreases.

April 10.—Less delirious. The jacket is drenched with sweat, and the patient has to be changed. Pulse large, soft, 88. Tongue coated white.

Cough rare; scanty sputa some of which is mucous and the rest preserves its yellow-brown color; but this latter portion scatters more readily than the evening previous. The respiratory movements are full and remarkably slow.

Large vesicular crepitation in front; behind it is finer and more abundant; bellows'-murmur more circumscribed and softer.—*Bryonia* two solutions.

The sweating continues the remainder of the day. The following night is a good one, and the delirium gradually ceases.

April 11.—Tongue coated white and moist; skin moist, without any great heat; pulse large, 76 to 80. No more delirium. The patient feels faint at the stomach, and desires to eat.

Cough less and less frequent; scarcely a little mucous expectoration, streaked with rusty phlegm.

Fine and copious *crepitans redux* in front and behind. The bellows'-sound continues slightly below the clavicle.—Continue *Bryonia.*

April 12.—The patient begs for food. Tongue coated and moist; pulse slow, soft, compressible.

Respiration harsh below the clavicle, with crepitant rattle perceptible only during the cough and at the close of a deep inspiration, not at all behind, where the respiratory murmur begins to become a little normal.—*Phosphorus* in solution.

April 13.—Two broths.—14. The harshness disappears gradually.—17. Had an epileptic fit last night, in consequence of which he remained in a state of apathy the whole of the 18th.

Discharged cured May 7th.

In this case the improvement commenced promptly after the exhibition of Bryonia, and the resolution took place very speedily.

Shortly after it had commenced, the patient was seized with an epileptic fit. Such attacks frequently recur in epileptic patients after an acute malady. I have seen this frequently after various acute diseases.

CASE 17.—*Compound pneumonia.*

Berthelot, aged 32 years, street-sweeper, of ordinary constitution, had fever and ague at the age of 19 years. This fever resisted a whole month to Quinine, and terminated in ascitis, which ceased in a fortnight. Since then his health had been good.

Last Friday, April 28th, while sweeping the street, he was taken sick and had to go home. He had scarcely laid down when he was taken with a violent chill which lasted for about an hour, and with a very severe dull headache. In proportion as the reaction set in, the headache became worse, a profuse discharge of blood took place from the nose and ears, and he felt so oppressed that he fancied he would choke, and had scarcely strength enough to call a neighbor from the next room to his assistance.

A physician was called who bled him profusely, after which the hæmorrhage ceased, the oppression gradually decreased, and was followed by a sharp, frequent cough with some bloody sputa.

During the night, he had a violent fever, cough with bloody sputa, and considerable difficulty of breathing. Next morning the physician had him sent to us, ward Sainte Cécile, No. 4.

April 29.—Flushed face, frontal headache, some nose-bleed; streaks of dried blood are seen from the external meatus auditorii to the lobules.

Tongue red, dry; intense thirst, skin dry and burning; pulse 112; cough frequent, bloody sputa mingled with air-vesicles on the surface.

Oppression; respiratory movements short, unequal; painful stitch in the side on a level with the left hypochondrium.

Percussed throughout its whole extent, the thorax

yields a good sound in front, on either side; but behind the sound is dull from the base to the top, and on both sides at the same time.

In front the respiratory murmur is feeble but distinct, without any other abnormal murmur. Behind, and on the left side, on a level with, and interiorly to the sub-spinal fossa, a very harsh bellows'-murmur is heard, which, at its limits, especially below, is mingled with a crepitant rattle that is heard only at the close of a deep inspiration. On the right side, and behind, there is a complete absence of respiratory murmur, even during ever so deep an inspiration. Bronchophony is quite manifest.—*Aconite* 6 in solution; water and sugar, two pitcherfuls.

April 30.—No new symptoms. The nosebleed has ceased. The tubular murmur extends over a larger surface of the thorax behind and on the left side. Behind and on the right side, there is a complete absence of respiratory murmur. The bloody sputa continues copious, but less shining than the day before.—*Bryonia* 18, two solutions.

In the evening, the oppression gets worse; the patient is very restless, and slightly delirious all night.

May 1.—The restlessness and the delirium are less. Intense headache, face bloated; tongue red and dry; a good deal of thirst.

Skin hot and dry. Pulse large, not very resisting, 104.

Stitch in the side equally acute and in the same region. Cough frequent, distressing; expectoration easier; bloody sputa more viscid and less filled with air-vesicles than on the previous days; some of the sputa looks rusty. The respiratory movements although short and rapid, seem to be performed with ease. The oppression is less.

The bellows'-murmur is less harsh behind and on the

left side, and is intermingled with a crepitant rattle which is no longer heard on its limits only. On the right side, where no murmur had been heard until now, a fine and copious crepitation is heard along the internal border of the scapula, with a slight bellows'-murmur during the expiration. Bronchophony on both sides.—Continue *Bryonia.*

May 2.—Spent a good night. About eleven o'clock the patient fell asleep, and woke at two o'clock in the morning covered with moisture.

In the morning, he had scarcely any headache, the face is no longer flushed, the tongue coated white and moist. Thirst moderate; skin warm, covered with copious perspiration (he has been changed three times). The pulse is large, soft, undulating, down to 80. Cough easy, rare, with copious expectoration of viscid and rusty sputa, some of which is blood-streaked. The breathing is full, easy; the stitch in the side is scarcely perceptible during the cough only.

Behind and on the left side, fine and copious *crepitans redux*, the tubular murmur and the bronchophony being scarcely perceived. On the right side, the murmur is more distinct and over a larger surface than the evening previous; crepitant rattle at the base.

The critical sweat ceases towards evening; the patient says he feels quite well.

May 3.—Tongue coated white and moist; no thirst. Skin natural; pulse large, soft, 76.

Cough rare, breathing easy; sputa not very copious, less viscid, partly vesicular, somewhat blood-streaked.

On the left side, the breathing begins to be normal. During the cough, and at the close of a deep inspiration, a fine crepitant rattle is heard, scattered over a surface. Slight distant bellows'-murmur.

On the right side, abundant and very fine *crepitans redux.*—*Bryonia* in solution.

May 4.—Skin natural; pulse 60.

Cough rare, saffron-colored, diffuse sputa, somewhat blood-streaked. *Bryonia* and *Sulphur* in alternation.

May 5.—Breathing on the left side normal; on the right side, the crepitans redux is only heard at the end of a deep inspiration.—*Bryonia* in solution; broth.

May 6.—Bryonia, and two broths.—Pulse 56.

May 7.—Bryonia, two spoonfuls; two broths, two soups. Pulse 52 to 56.

Discharged cured May 17th.

In this case we have to notice the bleeding resorted to on the first day. The Aconite which was administered on the second day, seems to have quieted the patient somewhat. On the third day, *Bryonia* was given. It was followed by a striking aggravation, after which the resolution gradually took place with rapidity; for on the fifth day, instead of having an exacerbation of the symptoms, the patient feels well. This compound pneumonia, which was an extensive and serious inflammation, was terminated happily and speedily. The pulse came down to 52.

CASE 18.—*Pneumonia of the left lung, upper lobe.*

Adnet, 29 years old, of the Republican guard, was admitted May 16th, 1848.

He is strong, sanguine, and has always enjoyed good health.

Last Saturday, May 14th, he was on duty, exposed to the rain all morning; about four in the afternoon he was seized with a chill, vertigo, and a violent pain in the loins which lasted until 10 o'clock. Then came the heat, an intense thirst, an intense headache with buzzing in the ears, and a seated pain in the præcordial region, which renders the breathing very difficult. Next morning he is moreover attacked with a frequent cough accompanied by serous and vesicular sputa which is somewhat blood-streaked.

May 16.—Was admitted to our hospital; the face is red and bloated. Intense frontal headache, with buzzing in the ears.

Tongue coated white and moist, thirst moderate.

Skin moderately warm. Pulse full, large, 116 to 120. Respiration anxious and frequent; stitch in the side not very acute during the ordinary respiratory movements, but very painful during the cough.

The cough is very frequent, distressing, followed by a sanguineous expectoration of a uniform red color, and very tenacious.

Percussion yields a dull sound behind and on the left side in the sub-spinous fossa, and in front, from the clavicle to the fourth rib. In this space, auscultation reveals crepitation with unequal bullæ, breaking in masses during a paroxysm of cough. Between second and third rib in front, the expirations are tubular. *Aconite* 6 in solution, two tumblerfuls; sugar and water two pitcherfuls.

May 17.—Same as yesterday. Skin continues moist. Pulse 116; sputa of a lighter color, more copious.—Water and sugar; *Bryonia* 12, two solutions.

Evening: The patient is very restless. Breathing very frequent, anxious, with distressing cough and scanty expectoration.

Pulse strong; skin less moist, intensely hot.

The whole night was spent in this condition, without any sleep.

May 18.—Headache less intense, and the expression of anguish less. The buzzing continues, and incommodes the patient a good deal.

Tongue coated white and moist; very little thirst. Pulse large, 100.

Breathing less frequent; the stitch, which in scarcely felt any more in its original locality, has changed to a sense of constriction at the base of the thorax, on the left side.

Cough frequent; easy and copious expectoration of viscid and rusty sputa, floating in the midst of a gum-like liquid, which fills the lower part of the vessel.

Dulness of sound in front and behind much less. Large masses of unequal crepitation in front, where the bellows'-murmur is less harsh. The murmur is heard in the sub-spinal fossa, where it had not been heard before.—*Bryonia* 12, two solutions.

May 19.—During the night the patient was restless, and the cough more frequent. The patient slept from two to four in the morning, and woke in perspiration; he had to be changed three times.

In the morning, Dr. Tessier only felt of his pulse which was down to 84; the patient says he feels quite well.— Continue Bryonia 12 and 24.

Copious nose bleed about noon. In the evening the buzzing ceases. Cough almost gone. The expectorated substance resembles a solution of gum mixed with vesicular serum.

May 20.—Spent a good night.—Headache almost gone. Temperature of the skin natural; cough rare; serous, scattering sputa. Pulse 72.

Crepitans redux in front and behind, perceived only at the end of a deep inspiration. Dulness of sound almost ceased.—*Bryonia in solution.*

May 21.—Unequal crepitant rattles scattered over a surface, at the end of a deep inspiration. Continue *Bryonia.* Pulse 60.

May 22.—Pulse 60. *Bryonia*, broth.

May 23.—Pulse 48 to 52. Bryonia 24, two broths.

May 24.—Pulse down to 44.—Two broths, a soup. Discharged cured May 27.

This case is conclusive as regards the efficacy of the treatment. Under the influence of Bryonia, the pulse came down to 44.

CASE 19.—*Pneumonia of the right lung.*

Hermanns, aged 35 years, admitted July 7th, 1848, ward St. Benjamin, No. 26.

This patient is of a thin and dry constitution, not very strong; is frequently attacked with pneumonia. Had the first attack when he was 20 years old, in Holland. The right lung was diseased. This attack was not very severe, and treated with emetics and cathartics; it was cured in four days; but he was not quite well until at the end of a month.

At the age of 30, in Paris, he had a second attack on the same lung, and remained three weeks in the hospital St. Antoine, with Dr. Kapeler. He was treated with venesections, cuppings, blisters, during the ten days that the real inflammation lasted.

At he age of 33, another attack, treated in the same manner. Was sick eight days, and recovered rapidly.

At the age of 34, in 1847, fourth attack, treated by Dr. Recurt with venesections and tartar emetic. This time the patient had to remain in bed for three weeks, laid up with fever, cough, rusty sputa and a stitch in the side, which disappears previous to the other symptoms at the end of a fortnight.

Between the attacks, Hermanns enjoyed good health, had neither a cold nor any other disease. These inflammations always set in in consequence of violent exertions, after working all night at his trade, cabinet-making. In this condition the least cold brought on the attack. This exposure is so certainly followed by the disease, that he asserts he can bring on an attack any time he chooses.

Last Tuesday, July 4th, after moving, and covered with perspiration, he drank cold water to quench his thirst. Immediately after he was taken sick, had a fever, but no chill; he expected his customary attack, and went to bed soon after a stitch in the right side in front was felt; he coughed, and spent a restless and sleepless night. Next morning he raised blood. In this condition he remained home without any treatment, except herb-tea.

On the 7th he was brought to the hospital.

In the evening he showed the following symptoms: Countenance expresses lowness of spirits; eyes dull, malar regions flushed; no headache.

Tongue dry, whitish in the middle, with red borders; thirst moderate.

Pulse quick, compressible, 120 beats. Skin hot and remarkably dry.

The patient in only comfortable when lying on the back.

Stitch in the side not very acute, behind and on the right side; the stitch is only felt during the cough.

Striking dyspnœa. The right side of the thorax remains unmoved during the act of respiration. On the right side the breathing is short, frequent, but regular.

Cough not frequent, not very fatiguing, and giving rise to a viscid, brick-colored expectoration.

Percussion yields a dull sound behind in the sub-spinal depression at the base of the thorax, extending outward as far as the axilla.

Auscultation reveals bronchial murmur in the sub-spinal fossa during an inspiration and expiration. Exteriorly, along the border of the scapula, we have an abundant and very fine crepitant rattle. Toward the inferior angle of the same bone, the crepitating bullæ are unequal, larger, less numerous.

This first examination, which showed the true character of the perceptible phenomena of this case, was instituted at 7 o'clock in the evening. The physician on duty bled the patient immediately after his admission, three basinfuls.—*Aconite* 12 in solution.

July 8.—No change except that the dyspnœa was much worse.—*Bryonia* two solutions.

At five in the evening, the patient became rather restless and flighty. The patient wants to go out.

July 9.—The night has been very restless, no sleep; the cough is very frequent.

In the morning the fever and the general symptoms are the same as on the previous days. The skin continues dry and parched.

Cough frequent; the patient raises with more ease a copious viscid sputa, rusty and having lost its former brick color; it is mixed with a little vesicular serum.

Dyspnœa intense; stitch in the side scarcely felt.

The bellows'-murmur is spread over a larger surface. It is perceived at the base of the chest and along the external border of the capsula. Along the inner border the murmur is less harsh.—Continue *Bryonia* 12.

July 10.—Pretty good night; not restless. About 10 o'clock in the evening a slight moisture shows itself on the thorax, in the face and on the upper limbs. The patient is henceforth quiet, but has no sleep.

In the morning, the face has lost its sinking expression; the malar region is no longer flushed.

The tongue is coated white and moist. Thirst more intense.

Skin dry, but of a mild temperature.

Pulse compressible, but fuller, down to 100.

Respiration full and easy.

Stitch in the side almost gone. Cough increases in frequency. The patient raises a rusty sputa, surrounded, at the bottom of the vessel, by a large quantity of vesicular serum.

Continued dulness of sound.

The bronchial respiration is not harsh on a level with the internal border of the spine of the scapula, and, during an inspiration, is intermingled with a few crepitating vesicles. Below and toward the axilla, it is scarcely heard at the end of an expiration. Crepitation is likewise heard in this space.—Continue *Bryonia.*

July 11.—The patient slept from one to four o'clock in the morning. On waking he has to discharge a large quantity of urine.

In the forenoon the skin is moist. Pulse down to 76 or 80.

The tubular murmur is limited to the roots of the bronchia. Any where else *crepitans redux.*

Less expectoration, scarcely colored; not much serum. Feels comfortable.—*Bryonia.*

July 12.—All over crepitans redux; the murmur is limited and distant.

Mucous expectoration, slightly mixed with air-vesicles. Continue *Bryonia.*

July 13.—Pulse 60. Distant murmur; crepitation only here and there, and not heard unless the patient coughs. Broth.

July 14.—Pulse 60. Murmur at the bronchial roots diminishing. In other parts the respiration becomes normal. *Phosphorus* in solution; two broths.

Convalescent; discharged July 18th in perfect health.

CASE 20.—*Pneumonia of the left side in the same patient.*

August 30th, Hermanns returns to the hospital, ward St. Benjamin.

Last night he was attacked with a dry cough an acute stitch in the left axilla, without any assignable cause. Went to bed, and, two hours after, was taken with wandering chills, alternating with flushes of heat. The cough continued all night, dry, fatiguing and painful. At daybreak the skin became slightly moist and he raised some blood-streaked phlegm.

On coming to the hospital, he showed the following symptoms: Face bloated, but not much headache.

Tongue dry, covered in the middle with a thin whitish coating, with red tip and edges. Intense thirst.

Skin warm, moist all over, and a few drops of sweat on the forehead.

Pulse large, soft, 112 to 116.

The oppression is not very great, the breathing hurried.

Cough frequent, painful, and followed by difficult expectoration of serous sputa, mixed with air-vesicles and slightly blood-streaked.

The stitch in the side is very distressing.

He is neither restless nor anxious, and does not feel very sick.

Percussion yields a rather dull sound below the left axilla in the space of four fingers'-breadth; and behind, the dulness is perceived on the same side, in the same space, in the sub-spinal fossa.

Below the axilla, complete absence of all respiratory murmur; behind, at the lower part of the scapula, an abundant crepitation is heard at the end of an inspiration, and a gentle, distant bellows'-murmur at the end of an expiration. Scarcely any bronchophony in these two regions.

In every other part of the chest the resonance is normal and the breathing natural, perhaps a little labored and somewhat harsh under the left clavicle.—Two pitcherfuls of sugar and water; two solutions of *Bryonia*.

Sept. 1.—Last night, about 6 o'clock, the skin, which had been moist, became dry, and remained so until morning.

Night pretty fair; the cough had been distressing and had kept the patient awake; he would have slept, if it had not been for the cough.

In the morning the skin was found moist and gently warm. Pulse soft and large, 112.

Cough frequent; sputa not very copious, rusty, viscid, without scarcely any serum of which it consisted almost entirely before.

Stitch in the side very acute; no dyspnœa properly speaking. The tubular murmur is more marked, harsher, spread over a larger surface. The crepitation is limited to the base of the lung, and is only heard during an attack of cough or a deep inspiration.

No respiratory murmur in the axilla.—Continue the same treatment.

Sept. 2.—Same as yesterday, almost. Pulse down to 96; the stitch is less painful and the cough less distressing; viscid and rusty sputa. Stethoscopic signs the same.

Sept. 3.—Slept two or three hours in the night, the cough being less frequent and less distressing.

In the morning the patient feels quite comfortable.

The face is no longer bloated; the thirst, which, until now, had been intense, is scarcely felt. Tongue coated white and moist.

Skin of the temperature of the breath. Pulse soft and compressible, down to 84.

Cough unfrequent; expectoration easy and copious, consisting partly of serous and vesicular sputa, partly of rusty sputa in small quantity.

The stitch in the side is almost gone; it is scarcely felt during the cough.

Continual dulness in the above mentioned spaces.

Under the axilla, an abundant crepitation is heard, with unequal vesicles. Behind it is heard from the spine of the scapula to the base of the lung, being of the same character. Bronchial respiration is not very distinct on a level with the sub-spinal depression; it is harsh and intense only on a level with the bronchial roots, where bronchophony is likewise distinctly heard.—*Bryonia* in solution; water and sugar.

In the afternoon a slight sweat breaks out.

Next night, sound sleep and rest.

Sept. 4.—Skin natural; pulse 68 to 72.

Cough rare, with serous and mucous sputa not very abundant. Crepitation and bellows'-murmur continue.—*Bryonia.*

Sept. 5.—Pulse 64. Now and then a little cough. Scanty serous and mucous expectoration. Crepitation disappears all over. The bellows'-murmur is still heard towards the middle portion of the inner border of the scapula.—*Phosphorus* 12, in solution.

Sept. 6.—The tubular murmur is less distinct.—Continue Phosphorus.

Sept. 7.—Tne respiratory murmur is heard in the whole extent of the inflamed lung. The bronchial respiration is scarcely heard.—Two broths.

Sept. 8, 9, 10.—*Bryonia,* one solution every day; the pulse comes down to 48 beats.

Sept. 12; discharged cured.

CASE 21.—*Compound pneumonia.*

July 10th, 1848, Lefèvre, blacksmith, aged 51 years, was admitted in the ward St. Benjamin No. 15.

This man was naturally feeble, and had been in bad health for the last ten years. Ten years ago he was attacked with pneumonia which was treated for about twelve days with venesections and tartar emetic, and was followed by a convalescence of a month's duration, at the end of which period the patient was able to resume his work. His health was not entirely restored; for ever since he had this disease he had remained subject to pulmonary catarrh, each attack of which was characterised by an obstinate cough, especially at night, and followed in the morning by a profuse mucous expectoration. These attacks recurred at irregular periods, and were altogether regulated by atmospheric influences, cold weather, rain &c.; they were never accompanied by fever, nor was the patient obliged to quit work during the attack.

But at the beginning of spring, and at the close of fall in every year, the attacks were always worse and the cough more distressing than at other times; and at these periods the expectoration was more copious, and a fever accompanied the attack, obliging the patient to keep his bed for eight or ten days, at the end of which period his health became good again, and he was able to return to his business. The patient had no other treatment during the attack than diet and herb-teas.

Last April, after having had a cough and fever for three or four days, as usual in the spring, this fever and cough became very intense, and the patient raised blood. A very painful stitch in the side attacked him, and the patient was treated for this *cold on the chest*, as it was termed, by Dr. Belhomme, doubtless with bleeding and tartar emetic. For about ten days the disease was very serious; and after the characteristic signs of pneumonia had been dispersed, his convalescence was still long and distressing, or, rather, he had never been perfectly restored to health. He lost flesh; his strength decreased from day to day; a slight fever, with heat, restlessness, and moisture in the morning, troubled him every night. His cough never ceased, and distressed the patient more particularly after a meal, even ever so slight; it came in paroxysms which terminated in the raising of a whitish mucus. Every morning, on waking and after the sweat ceased, the paroxysms of cough lasted longer and were more distressing than during the remainder of the day, and he then raised a yellowish matter.

While troubled with this chronic malady, for which he did not pursue any treatment, and during which he even pursued his ordinary work as much as he was able, the cough and fever suddenly became continual, and he had to go to bed. This was on the fourth of July. The cough, which had generally been loose, suddenly became dry, except that, on the first day; he raised a few strings of pure mucus; on the second day he raised streaks of blood; and this continued until the expectoration looked altogether bloody. At the same time a constrictive pain, which was not very violent at first, but increased in intensity, was felt all around the chest on a level with the false ribs, and imparted a sensation as if an iron band had been applied round this part of the body. A distressing dyspnœa developed itself with the other symptoms, and, after having suffered in this way for six days, he applied fcr admission in the hospital, on the 10th of July, where he showed the following symptoms:

Countenance worn out; striking emaciation; livid color of the skin. Marked debility; inability to sit up.

No headache. Tongue coated white, moist, with red edges. Thirst moderate.

Skin dry, warm all over, except on the forehead and in the palms of the hands, which are moist.

Pulse small, tense, 96 to 100.

Dyspnœa intense; breathing short and frequent. The patient complains more particularly of the feeling of oppression and the circular constriction round the epigastric region.

The cough is constant and painful. Expectoration viscid, homogeneous, rusty, strongly adhering to the bottom of the vessel, without any admixture of serum.

Percussion does not yield any dulness of sound any where in the whole extent of the thorax. Behind and below, on a level with the lower angle of the scapula, the sound is a little dull on either side; but this dulness is not complete.

Auscultation furnishes the following signs: below the clavicles, anteriorly to either side of the thorax, the respiration is not disturbed either as regards the rhythm or the murmurs, it is harsh behind; bronchial bellows'-murmur on both sides, along the inner border of the scapula, harsh on the right side, less on the left. Sub-crepitant rattle abundant, moist at the base of the left lung during an ordinary inspiration; on the right side, the crepitation is very fine, and heard only during the cough. Diffuse bronchophony on both sides.—*Bryonia* 12 and *Carbo veget.* 12, in solution, alternately; water and sugar.

July 11.—Same as yesterday except the following modification:

Copious sputa during the night, but viscid and rusty.

Pulse less tense, 100.

Skin less dry. The hands are moist. The face is covered with sweat.

Stethoscopic signs the same.—*Bryonia* 12 and 24, two solutions.

At two o'clock in the afternoon, a slight moisture broke out all over. At 6 in the evening, the constriction was much less; the respiration is fuller, less hurried; oppression still very considerable.

July 12.—No sleep. The skin remains moist, but not much sweat. Three copious diarrhœic stools during the night.

In the morning, the countenance has a good expression. Feels comfortable.

Tongue coated white and moist. No thirst. Skin moist, of a mild temperature. Pulse 68.

The constriction is only felt during the cough and a deep inspiration.

Respiration still frequent. Dyspnœa continues.

Cough rare; scattering sputa like dissolved gum, mixed with frothy serum. No dulness.

Bronchial murmur scarcely heard behind and on the left side; sub-crepitant rattle from the sub-spinal depression to the base of the lung. On the right side, continued harsh bellows'-murmur with diffuse bronchophony; abundant crepitation of large vesicles below.—*Bryonia* 12, two solutions, *Sulphur* 6, in alternation.

July 13.—Frequent cough in the night.

The cough continues during the day. Profuse mucous vesicular sputa. Dyspnœa.

Scattering crepitation right and left. Bellows'-murmur less harsh and mingled with a crepitant rattle at the close of an inspiration on the right side; bronchophony. —Continue *Bryonia* and *Sulphur.*

July 14.—Cough, with mucous expectoration.—Two broths.

July 15.—Less cough.—*Sulphur* 12.

July 20.—Little cough; mucous and frothy sputa. Respiratory murmur normal on the left side, except at the base of the lung, where some crepitation continues to be heard. Mucous rattle on the right side. The bellows'-murmur has ceased.——An allowance.——Discharged cured July 24.

CASE 22.—*Pneumonia of the right lung.*

Escaille, aged 35 years, weaver, of a feeble constitution and nervous temperament, admitted July 11th, 1848, ward St. Benjamin No. 28.

This man had injoyed good health until 1836, when he was attacked with a quartan intermittent, while in garrison in the South of France; he remained sick for six months, and, at the close of this period, he was moreover attacked with ascites, which finally left him, together with the fever, under the use of quinine and diuretics. He was perfectly cured, and has never had another paroxysm since.

Three weeks ago he commenced to complain of a bad taste in his mouth, with loss of appetite and aversion to food. Every morning, on rising, he was taken with nausea; the least thing he ate in the day-time oppressed his stomach, and in the evening he was distressed by a feeling of malaise, uneasiness and restlessness, without any appearance of fever; these symptoms disappeared at night, and he slept profoundly. Diet and cooling beverages stopped the nausea and the bad taste in the mouth in about a week; but the malaise, the loss of appetite, and the weakness continued and even grew worse.

On the fourth of July the feeling of weariness in the extremities became so great that the patient had scarcely left his bed, when he was obliged to return to it. From this moment he commenced to cough and to complain of a slight stitch in the right hypochondrium, with a few wandering chills now and then in the course of the day. In the evening, he was suddenly seized with a violent chill, commencing in the loins and back, and gradually spreading over the rest of the body. This chill, which lasted about an hour and convulsed the extremities and jaws, made the patient apprehensive of a return of his former disease. But a reaction having speedily developed itself, with a seated headache in the forehead, and more particularly with oppression of breathing, a violent cough and a stitch in the side that tormented him all night; and not seeing any sweat, he sent for a physician the next morning, who told him that he was suffering with pulmonary catarrh, and ordered him a bottle of Seltzers' water, and a cataplasm in the region of the stitch.

From the 5th to the 10th of July the oppression and fever continued and grew worse. On the sixth, the cough, which had been dry until then, was followed by a little blood-streaked mucus. No treatment was pursued except that above mentioned, cataplasms and a decoction of marsh-mallow.

July 11th, having spent a very bad night, on account of the cough and the oppression which had become excessive, he was taken to the hospital.

Two hours after his arrival, he showed the following symptoms:

The patient lies on his back; complete prostration of strength; the patient is wearied by the questions that are put to him, and is scarcely able to answer yes or no. Countenance animated, with flushes on the malar region. Little or no headache.

Tongue dry, wih a red tip and red borders, covered in the middle with a dry and brownish coating. Thirst intense, he asks for drink all the time.

Skin dry, with a stinging heat.

Pulse small, 120 to 124.

Stitch in the side, scarcely painful and having shifted from the hypochondrium to the right posterior thoracic region, toward the base of the lung; it is only when coughing that the pain becomes acute.

Marked oppression. Breathing short and frequent.

Cough rare; he had expectorated only three times, a rusty, viscid sputa, strongly adhering to the bottom of the vessel, and not containing any air-vesicles; behind and on the right side the sound is completely dull from the spine of the scapula to the base of the lung.

Auscultation reveals a feeble respiration at the anterior portion of the thorax. Behind, in the sub-spinal depression, a little crepitation is heard at the end of an inspiration. Below, no rattle, but an intense tubular murmur is heard during an inspiration and expiration.—*Aconite* 6, and *Bryonia* 6 in solution, alternately.

Saw the patient again between 11 o'clock and midnight; he is very restless and prays to be relieved of the oppression that suffocates him.

July 12.—In the morning, we discover a slight remission in the symptoms. The dyspnœa is less; the pulse, skin, cough and the stethoscopic signs are the same.—Water and sugar, three pitcherfuls; Bryonia 6 and 12, two solutions.

At 7 in the evening, general aggravation of the symptoms. Countenance animated; restlessness and oppression are excessive; cough very frequent. The pulse, which had been small and tense, had become full, 116 to 120.

The cough had been increasing in frequency all night, Abundant saffron-colored and viscid sputa, with a little lighter-colored, scattering and vesicular sputa floating upon it.

July 13.—Face continues animated with flushed cheeks; perspiration on the forehead and on the wings of the nose. Tongue red at the borders, moist and covered with a whitish mucus. Thirst intense; no headache.

Skin hot and dry, but the heat is no longer stinging; perspiration in the palms of the hands. Pulse large, 100. Stitch in the side almost gone, scarcely felt when coughing.

Respiration fuller and less frequent; the respiratory movements are not embarassed; the patient considers himself *saved*, because, says he, *he is able to breathe.*

Cough very frequent; the spittoon is half full of the previously described sputa.

Complete dulness of sound behind, especially low down.

Tubular murmur only during an expiration, along the inner border of the scapula. Diffuse bronchophony in the same space. Broncho-egophony quite low down, where the dulness of sound is perfect.

During an inspiration, the *crepitans redux* is heard in voluminous masses.

Harsh respiration and rhonchus in the subspinal fossa.—Two pitcherfuls of water and sugar; two solutions of *Bryonia*, 12, 24.

It was not till this day that the patient was able to relate the circumstances of his previous illness, which have been mentioned at the beginning.

July 14.—Slept and perspired last night. Skin warm and moist; breathing free. Pulse 76. Cough frequent and easy; profuse mucous sputa containing air-vesicles. Bellows'-murmur, *crepitans redux*; broncho-egophony at the base of the thorax. Dulness of sound in this region.—Continue *Bryonia*.

July 15.—Pulse 60.—*Bryonia* 12.

July 16.—Pulse 44.—*Bryonia*.

July 17.—Pulse 40.—*Bryonia*; an allowance. The stethoscopic signs disappear. Discharged cured July 21st.

CASE 23.—*Pneumonia of the left side.*

Baudoin, aged 26 years, of a robust constitution, was admitted July 14th, 1848, in the ward St. Benjamin, No. 29.

Last Sunday, July 9th, he was obliged to walk to Clichy, and was exposed to the rain for two hours. He had to keep his wet clothes on until late in the evening. Next morning he rose with a feeling of soreness and weariness, headache, complete loss of appetite. In the night following he was restless, had no sleep, and on Tuesday morning he had not yet left his bed when he was taken with a violent chill and an acute stitch in the side, that prevented him from breathing. The remainder of the day he had a violent fever. In the night following he commenced to cough and complained of great difficulty of breathing.

July 12.—Fever, frequent cough, sanguineous expectoration, stitch in the side, oppression. He was bled copiously, and eight leeches were applied to the stitch.

July 13.—Same symptoms. No change of treatment.

July 14.—Came to the hospital, sense of prostration, lies on the back.

Dull headache; tongue moist and moving about easily; thirst moderate.

Skin warm and dry; pulse large, 116 to 120. Breathing frequent and harsh; the patient complains of oppression, and of a stitch opposite the left nipple, that renders his cough distressing and fatiguing. Sputa scattering, of a greenish-red color. Thorax sounds well in front; dulness in the left posterior portion, and below the left axilla. Intense bellows'-murmur in the subspinal fossa, less intense below, where it is mingled with abundant mucous rattle.—*Bryonia* 12, 24, two solutions.

July 15.—No sleep in the night, restless; frequent cough.

During the remainder of the day the symptoms remain the same as yesterday. The countenance is expressive of prostration. The sputa, which remains of a greenish-red color and scatters, is less.—Continue *Bryonia.*

July 16.—No sleep at night. The cough has become very frequent, but is less distressing; less oppression; raised a good deal in the night; the spittoon is filled with a sputa, that looks the same and scatters as on the preceding days; it is mixed with a little yellow, vesicular mucus.

Pulse large, soft, 100. Tongue coated white, moist, moving easily; no headache. Temperature of the skin almost natural. General moisture.

No stitch in the side during an ordinary inspiration; it is still felt a little during the cough. Dulness of sound; mucous rattle throughout the whole extent of the posterior portion of the thorax. Bellows-murmur without harshness, and only heard during an expiration. Continue *Bryonia.*

Such is the condition of the patient in the morning. During the day, cough and expectoration continue the same. The moisture on the skin changes to sweat, and about noon the patient had to be changed.

At six o'clock in the evening, he says he feels pretty comfortable.

July 17.—Refreshing sleep from midnight until four o'clock. The sweating continues.

In the morning the tongue is moist and coated white.

Pulse large, soft, 80 to 84. Skin feels natural.

No dyspnœa; cough rare; scanty mucous expectoration, filled with air-vesicles.

Dulness, *crepitans redux*. Bronchial bellows'-murmur during an expiration.—Continue *Bryonia*.

In the evening, return of the heavy frontal headache. Pulse vibratory, rises to 100.—*Aconite* 12 in solution.

July 18.—Sleepless and restless nights. The patient had been flighty, and had complained of his headache all the time.

In the morning, frontal headache; hot skin; pulse 96, undulating; cough and expectoration almost gone; stethoscopic signs the same as yesterday.—*Bryonia* 24 and 12, two solutions.

At 8 o'clock in the evening, had a copious nosebleed.

July 19.—Very good night.

In the morning the patient feels very smart; desires a broth; pulse down to 64. Skin normal. Mucous expectoration.

Dulness of sound, mingled with a little crepitation and bronchial murmur.—Diet. *Bryonia* 12 in solution.

July 20.—Two broths. Dulness and murmur decrease.

July 21.—The patient leaves his bed.—Two broths, a soup; discharged cured July 24.

CASE 24.—*Pneumonia of the right side.*

Togné, glazier, 42 years old, tall, thin, dry, and with a constitution shattered by misery and toil, had been subject since his childhood to temporary indispositions, which lasted two or three days, and were characterized by a sense of weariness and a little fever, and yielded to rest. They generally set in in consequence of hard work or abuse of liquor. Except these indispositions, he has never had any long or serious illness that required the interference of art. He has never had a rheumatic disease, although he has often taken cold while in perspiration. In such a case he felt somewhat stiff and sore in the limbs, but these symptoms passed off again after sweating.

Sept. 14th, he took cold, and feeling very thirsty, he went on a drinking bout with his companions in order to dissipate his unpleasant feelings. At 11 at night he was playing cards, when he was taken with a violent chill and a shrill and frequent cough, that lasted all night.

In the morning complete remission of the symptoms and cessation of the cough. He only felt tired. Feeling so much better, he resumed his work.

Sept. 15th, in the evening, he was taken with another chill, which was soon followed by heat, and cough in the morning, with sweat and a little watery expectoration.

Saturday morning: apyrexia, but greater lassitude than the day before, and wandering pains at the right shoulder and arm, in the left hypochondrium and in the loin; in spite of this feeling of illness he goes to his work.

Sept. 16th, about nine in the evening, he is again taken with a chill, which was more violent than the last one, followed by fever, dry and fatiguing cough, dyspnœa, and a painful stitch in the left hypochondrium. He keeps his bed, experiences a slight remission of the symptoms in the day-time, and a violent aggravation in the night from Sept. 17 to 18; on this day he was admitted in the ward St. Benjamin, No. 20.

Sept. 18, in the evening: Marked prostration; the patient is unable to sit up; lies on his back.

Countenance sunken, eyes dull, and slightly jaundiced color of the sclerotica.

Tongue dry; intense thirst. Anxiety and slight restlessness.

Skin very hot and dry; pulse 120, rather hard.

Respiration difficult, anxious, intermittent.

Cough almost constant, fatiguing, and giving rise to a watery, vesicular, blood-streaked expectoration.

Dulness on the right side, below the nipple, in front, and also behind, below the sub-spinal fossa. Any where else the thorax yields normal sounds.

In front, low down and on the right side, complete absence of the respiratory murmur; behind, at the inner portion of the sub-spinal fossa, a harsh and dry bellows'-murmur.

The patient does not exactly complain of a painful stitch in any particular locality; he only complains of a general painful constriction around the lower part of the thorax from one side to the other, especially during the cough.—Two pitcherfuls of sugar and water; *Aconite* 6, and *Bryonia* 12 in alternation.

Sept. 19.—Restless night; oppression and anxiety worse; delirium has set in, during which the patient rose twice.—Mustard-plasters to the feet.

In the morning, same as yesterday, except the delirium, which had set in. The face is pale and looks sad; the patient is morose, frightened. Sputa more abundant, tougher, slightly viscid, and entirely bloody.—*Bryonia* 12, two solutions.

In the evening, about 5 o'clock, the delirium and restlessness are still worse. While raising the patient in bed and placing him in a sitting position, his forehead becomes covered with a cold sweat and he faints away for a short time.

Sept. 20.—The restlessness, anxiety and delirium have been less violent than the preceding night. The patient has made no attempt to escape.

In the morning: continued delirium, the prostration

seems less; the face is less pale, the eye more animated.

Tongue dry and red; thirst intense.

Skin dry and parched, hot; pulse rapid, small, 116 to 120.

Oppression the same. The breathing is short, unequal, frequent. The patient complains of a painful spot under the left breast; the pain is increased very sensibly by the cough.

Cough very frequent but easier; profuse expectoration of bloody sputa, mixed with a frothy serum.

The bellow's-sound is replaced posteriorly, at the base of the lung, by a scattered crepitant rattle; but it has ascended to the top of the lung, and it is now heard in the sub-spinal fossa. In front, under the clavicle, the respiratory murmur is simply exaggerated. *Bryonia* and *Phosphorus* 12 in alternation.

In the evening the pulse becomes full and large, but remains compressible 116.

Sept. 21.—During the night, the restlessness and delirium increased until midnight; the patient attempted to escape. After midnight he became quiet and coughed less; he perspired and had to be changed once.

In the morning, the delirium continues; but he was cheerful instead of morose. The patient wants to know what he owes his physician, and desires to leave.

His strength returns; he is able to sit up in bed, and his features no longer depict sadness nor lowness of spirits. The eye has become quick and sparkling.

The tongue continues red and dry. Thirst more moderate.

The dyspnœa is much less, also the stitch in the side. The breathing is fuller and more regular.

Cough still frequent. Expectoration more easy; bloody sputa very profuse, not very tenacious, with a large quantity of frothy serum floating upon it.

The dulness has decreased at the base of the lung in

front, below the nipple, where the respiratory murmur reappears. Posteriorly, scattered crepitation towards the base of the lung. The bellows'-murmur in the sub-spinal fossa is less harsh. When coughing, a few large moist vesicles are heard to crepitate. Intense bellows'-murmur in the sub-spinal fossa.—*Bryonia* 12, two solutions.

Sept. 22.—Night middling fair; delirious and restless. The day is pretty much the same as yesterday. Pulse down to 108.—Continue *Bryonia*.

Sept. 23.—Copious sweat all night; the patient had to be changed four times.

The merry delirium continues. He asks for his bill and wants to leave.

Tongue coated white and moist; thirst moderate.

Skin moist all day; has to be changed twice. Pulse soft, compressible, 84.

Breathing easy; the stitch has ceased.

Cough frequent, with copious expectoration of the same kind as yesterday.

Same stethoscopic signs.—*Bryonia* and *Belladonna* 12 in solution, alternately.

Sept. 24.—The delirium continues. Last night the patient slept well.

Pulse large, soft, 84. Skin natural.

Cough easy, pretty frequent. Profuse expectoration which is less bloody, more viscid, mixed with vesicular serum.—*Belladonna* and *Arsenic* 12 in solution, alternately.

Sept. 25.—Continued delirium. No thirst. Temperature of the skin natural. Pulse 64.

Abundant *crepitans redux* below the sub-spinal fossa. The bellows'-murmur in the super-spinal fossa continues. —Same treatment.

Sept. 26.—No delirium. The patient desires to eat. —Pulse 56.

A little mucous expectoration.

Crepitans redux less abundant. The bellows'-murmur continues.—*Sulphur* 24; broth.

Sept. 27.—The murmur gradually disappears the next three days.—Two broths.—The strength returns very speedily; pulse remains at 56. Discharged cured Oct. 5th, 1848.

CASE 25.—*Pneumonia of the right side.*

Pot, porter, 36 years old, of an athletic constitution, was admitted in the ward St. Benjamin, No. 16, on the 28th of September, 1848.

The day previous he had worked hard all day, and had several times exposed himself to a cool draught of air while in perspiration. Towards evening he felt stiff and weary in his limbs, and had to quit work. As soon as he had lain down in bed, he was seized with a violent chill that shook the whole body for about an hour, and caused the teeth to chatter. After the chill a fever gradually set in, and the whole night the patient was tormented by an unquenchable thirst and a burning heat that rendered all covering intolerable.

This morning a stitch in the side on a level with and a little below the right breast. From the first, it was a seated, stitching pain, accompanied by oppression and cough. A physician was called, who at once advised him to go to the hospital.

An hour after his admission, Pot exhibits the following symptoms:

Face animated, bloated; acute frontal headache; he lies on the right side, the only side on which he is able to lie comfortably.

Tongue moist, covered with a whitish coating; thirst intense.

Skin burning. Pulse strong, 120.

Stitch in the side, which is painful only during an inspiration, when the patient is lying on the affected side, very unpleasant in any other position, and aggravated by pressure.

Not much dyspnœa. Breathing hurried. Only the inspirations are short and imperfect.

Cough rare. The spittoon contains a little blood-streaked, serous, vesicular expectoration.

The thorax, percussed with care, yields a normal sound, except behind, below and on the right side, where the sound is slightly dull.

Auscultation discloses a clean respiratory murmur on the left side, normal in front and behind. On the right side, in front and under the clavicle, the respiration is puerile; behind it is somewhat exaggerated in the sub-spinal fossa. From the spine of the scapula to the base of the thorax on the same side, there is a complete absence of respiratory murmur even during a deep inspiration.—Three pitcherfuls of water and sugar.—Two solutions of *Aconite* 6.

Sept. 29.—Moist all night; four copious diarrhœic stools; red urine with sediment.

In the morning: bloated countenance; intense supra-orbital headache.

Tongue coated white, humid; thirst intense.

Same position in bed.

Skin moist, very hot, but not pungent.

Pulse strong, 116 to 120.

Cough more frequent than the day previous, painful. Serous, bloody sputa. Oppression, hurried breathing.

Dulness behind, below and on the right side; fine crepitation in the same space, heard in masses.—Same beverage. *Bryonia* 12, two solutions.

Sept. 30.—The perspiration and diarrhœa have continued all night, with sleeplessness, but no restlessness.

Otherwise the symptoms are the same, except the cough which increases in frequency, and the expectoration, which has changed in color and consistence.

4*

The expectoration, which is scanty, yellow, viscid, resembles apricot-sauce.

Pulse down to 108 to 112, but continues strong and full. The dulness which was at first limited to the lower portion of the thorax, is heard over a larger surface. In the sub-spinal fossa the sound is dull. Tubular murmur without rattle quite low down; fine and abundant crepitation above, towards the upper portion of the lung.—Continue *Bryonia*, and same beverage.

Oct. 1.—The sweat and diarrhœa continue. Red urine with sediment.

The stitch is less. Dyspnœa more violent; the difficulty of breathing is very distressing to the patient. The breathing, however, is not any more hurried than the evening previous. Pulse 108. Skin continues moist.

Complete dulness in the whole of the posterior portion of the right side of the thorax. Fine crepitation in the super-spinal fossa, and in the space below, harsh tubular murmur, without rattle.—Two pitcherfuls of water and sugar. *Bryonia* and *Sulphur* 12 in solution, alternately.

Between 7 and 8 o'clock in the evening, a copious nose-bleed sets in.

In the night, the patient has a few naps and alternate waking spells. The patient had to get up three or four times on account of his diarrhœa.

Oct. 2.—Countenance natural, no headache.

Tongue coated white and moist; thirst moderate.

Skin hot; no sweat. Pulse large, soft, 96.

The stitch in the side is only felt during the cough. Oppression and hurriedness of breathing.

Cough increases in frequency; easy expectoration of the same color, but less tough, and more vesicular and transparent.

Dulness of sound the same.

Tubular murmur less dry and harsh in the sub-spinal fossa, and below, intermingled with a little scattered crepitation at the end of an inspiration and during the cough. On a level with the super-spinal fossa, and especially towards the internal border of the scapula, bronchial respiration intermingled with moist rattle. —Two pitcherfuls of water and sugar. *Sulphur* in solution.

Oct. 2.—Slept well in the night; had to rise at midnight, on account of the diarrhœa.

Cough rare; scanty expectoration of a serous mucus. Skin natural. Pulse 64.

Dulness of sound; bronchial murmur only heard during an expiration. General crepitation during a common respiration.—Water and sugar. *Bryonia* and *Sulphur* 12, alternately.

Oct. 4.—Same symptoms: tubular respiration during an expiration; less *crepitans redux*. Pulse 56 to 60. Same beverage. *Bryonia* 24.

Oct. 5.—Pulse 44. *Bryonia*; two broths.

Oct. 6.—Pulse 44.—Two broths.

Oct. 7.—Gradual disappearance of all the stethoscopic signs. Discharged cured Oct. 14th, 1848.

CASE 26.—*Pneumonia of the left side.*

Corsin, aged 43 years, rag-picker, had small-pox at the age of ten years, and served in Africa where he was for a long time laid up with fever and ague. Since his return in France he has always felt well. Towards the end of last August he commenced to complain of malaise and weakness, so that he was unable to work with the same vigor as previously. This state lasted for about a month, during which period he remained without any kind of treatment. On the 21st of September, after a long walk and a severe fatigue, during which he had perspired a good deal, he took off his clothes, and was suddenly attacked by a chill, followed soon after by heat and a little perspiration. At the same time his breathing was embarrassed, he coughed a good deal, and on the following morning, he raised a little blood.

Sept. 23 he entered the ward St. Benjamin, No. 18.

Skin warm like his breath; tongue covered with a whitish coating; thirst intense; pulse middling full, 100.

No stitch in the side, but the breathing was embarrassed by a sense of constriction of the base of the thorax, on the left side.

Cough rare; easy expectoration of rusty sputa in small quantity, and very viscid.

No respiratory murmur in the whole of the left side, except behind, towards the middle of the axillary border of the scapula, where a slight bellows'-murmur is heard, accompanied by crepitation, as often as the patient coughs or draws a long breath.

The thorax sounds well above and below the space where the tubular murmur and the rattle are heard. Here percussion yields a dull sound over a surface of about three inches sideways.—*Aconite* and *Bryonia* in solution, alternately; water and sugar.

Sept. 24.—Had a good night. The temperature of the skin remained the same, without any actual perspiration; cough and fever the same. In the morning, the symptoms were the same.—*Bryonia* in solution.

Sept. 25.—Tongue coated white and moist; pulse soft, undulating, 92.

Skin moist. The patient has to be changed three times.

Scarcely any difficulty of breathing. Cough decreases in frequency. A little viscid, rusty sputa, mixed with a little whitish mucus.

The respiratory murmur is heard in front of the thorax, and behind below the stitch; in this region a faint murmur and crepitation in large masses are heard. Dulness of sound circumscribed.—*Bryonia* 12.

Sept. 26.—Skin natural; pulse 72. No cough; mucous expectoration.

Less *crepitans redux*.—*Bryonia*.

Sept. 27.—Feels perfectly well. A little more crepitation at the end of a deep inspiration or during the cough.—*Phosphorus* in solution; two broths.

Sept. 28.—Two broths and soups.

Sept. 29.—The same. Discharged Oct. 2, 1848.

CASE 27.—*Compound pneumonia.*

Oct. 14th, 1848, Mrs. Bizet, a day-servant, aged 69 years, was admitted in the ward Sainte Anné, No. 4. She had a sound and strong constitution, had never been very sick, and had been free from accidents or infirmities until recently.

Yesterday, Oct. 13th, without any assignable cause, she was seized with a chill which lasted about two hours; it was not very severe, and was followed by moderate heat and a violent oppression of breathing.

In the evening, she had another chill, accompanied with a stitching pain on a level with the false ribs of the right side, a dry cough, not very frequent, and aggravating the pain, and finally dyspnœa. Soon after she felt hot and perspired. This condition lasted all night without any aggravation. Next morning the patient felt a little better, except the oppression, and she came to the hospital Oct. 14th.

An hour after her admission, she showed the following symptoms:

Lies any way; face pale and slight circumscribed redness of the malar region; eyes sparkling but moist; a little headache; lips and tongue dry; thirst intense. Had not perspired for the last three days; moderate heat and dryness of the skin. Pulse frequent, but not hard, from 100 to 104.

Violent dyspnœa, unpleasant sensation of heaviness over the whole thorax, and stitching pain on a level with the lower extremity of the sternum which is aggravated by cough and by a deep inspiration.

Cough dry, not very frequent; it excites a feeling of roughness in the fauces, which is followed by nausea and a momentary bitterness in the mouth, that disappears again as soon as the patient drinks something.

Percussion yields a marked dulness of sound at the lower and posterior portion of both sides of the thorax; on the right side, from the sub-spinal fossa to the base of the lung; on the left side it is only felt over a space of about four fingers'-breadth, quite low down at the base. Any where else, the resonance is normal.

Auscultation reveals a very harsh bellows'-murmur on the right side along the inner border of the scapula, from its spine to the lower angle; from the boundaries of this murmur towards the axilla, an abundant crepitation is heard. On the left side, in the space which corresponds to the dulness of sound, the respiratory murmur is not heard at all during the ordinary respiration; but during the cough, or at the end of a deep inspiration, large masses of a fine crepitant rattle strike upon the ear.—Two pitcherfuls of water and sugar; *Bryonia* 12 in solution; an emollient injection.

Oct. 15.—Bad night. The cough, which had been of moderate frequency until now, had been frequent and distressing until morning. Towards morning the patient had expectorated a little liquid serum; had had two copious stools; urine with a sediment. In the forenoon, same symptoms as last night; except that the pulse is full, soft, down to 84.—*Bryonia* 12, two solutions.

About three in the afternoon, a slight moisture is seen on the skin, and continues during the whole of next night, during which the patient rests; she has to be changed, and discharges a large quantity of red, sedimentous urine.

Oct. 16.—Feels quite comfortable. Countenance has a natural expression. Tongue moist and coated white; no thirst; neither headache nor nausea.

Temperature of the skin normal; pulse soft, compressible, down to 68.

Breathing free and easy, although she still complains of a dull sense of constriction over the whole thorax, especially around the false ribs. The stitching pain behind the sternum has ceased.

No cough, no expectoration.

Dulness of sound in the above-mentioned space.

The bellows'-murmur on the right side has become fainter and more distant; a crepitant rattle is heard on its limits, and likewise on the left side at the base of the lung, only when coughing.—*Bryonia* in solution; broth.

Oct. 17.—The patient desires to eat. Pulse slow and soft, 64.

Dulness continues, bellows'-murmur faint and distant, with scattered crepitation behind and on the right side; on the left side no abnormal murmur, the respiratory murmur is heard again.—*Bryonia* 24, three spoonfuls; broth.

Oct. 18.—Pulse slow, compressible, down to 52.

Bellows'-murmur scarcely heard.—Continue *Bryonia*; two broths and a soup.

On the following days the resolution became perfect; discharged cured Oct. 31st, 1848.

The cases which have been reported so far, seemed to me to appeal so eloquently to the judgment of the reader, that I have not deemed it necessary to offer any comment.

The sinking of the pulse after the exhibition of Bryonia has been seen. This phenomenon occurs almost regularly. The sinking is generally less when Phosphorus is given either after, or alternately with, Bryonia.

CASE 28.—*Pneumonia of the right side.*

Lucas, 44 years old, shoemaker, admitted on the 18th of Oct., 1848, ward St. Benjamin, No. 18.

The patient had an attack of pleurisy in 1824; he is not subject to colds, enjoys good health in general, is strong and has a good constitution. Eight days ago, after moving, he exposed himself to a cold draught while drenched with sweat; he felt this exposure keenly. During the three subsequent days, he did not experience any untoward symptom. But on the third day, having gone to bed early, he was seized with a violent chill towards midnight, and had cold sweats which lasted until morning. At the same time he felt a headache, a pain in the side, dyspnœa, and was attacked with a cough that aggravated the stitch in the side, and which he sought to suppress on this account; he complained of intense thirst and general weariness. During the following five days the symptoms became worse, but the patient declined treatment.

On the 19th of Oct., the day after his admission to the hospital, he showed the following symptoms:

Skin warm and dry; pulse frequent; thirst intense; tongue covered from the tip to the root with a whitish coating; mouth sticky, with bitter taste; costiveness since he was first taken sick; copious discharge of urine; frontal headache; slight icterus, particularly marked on the cunjunctivæ. Moderate anxiety; stitch in the whole right side of the thorax, going from before backwards, and particularly painful at the base of the thorax; cough frequent, followed by scanty expectoration of gummy sputa that adheres to the vessel, is filled with air vesicles on the surface, and mixed with a viscid substance of a yellow-brown color.

Had to be changed three times during the night; the sweat was cold, according to the patient's statement.

Marked dulness at the summit of the thorax, posteriorly, on the right side; it continues alike as far as the lower angle of the scapula, and decreases from this point to the base of the chest.

Auscultation reveals in the supraspinal fossa a bronchial murmur, mingled with a fine crepitant rattle in the whole upper part of the lung. From the spine of the scapula to the lower angle of this bone, we have bronchial bellows'-murmur, bronchophony, and a little crepitation only around the space where the murmur is most strongly heard. Low down the murmur disappears gradually. At the base there is neither murmur nor crepitation.

On the left side the sound is clear, respiration puerile. —*Bryonia* 12 in solution, and two pitcherfuls of water and sugar.

Oct. 20.—Pulse less frequent; skin continues hot and dry; intense thirst; tongue coated white; mouth sticky, bitter, urine copious and frequent; icterus the same; no anguish; oppression is only felt when the patient is placed in a sitting posture; cough nearly as frequent as the day before, dry, hacking, short; expectoration of various kinds, vesicular and ropy, or adhering to the vessel and light colored, or some of the color of an apricot. No sweat in the night or during the day.

Percussion.—Dulness of sound as yesterday; scarcely perceptible from the lower angle of the scapula downwards. Bronchial bellows'-murmur, and bronchophony in the supra-spinal fossa, with unequal crepitation; in the sub-spinal fossa, the bellows'-sound is intense, the bronchophony very loud; unequal large vesicles crepitate over the whole space of this fossa. Below the lower angle the respiration is heard easily; it is louder than in a normal condition, but without any particular murmurs.—*Bryonia* 12 and 24, two solutions; beverage the same.

Oct. 21.—Pulse regular, normal; skin moist, sweat slightly warm, like the breath; thirst pretty violent; tongue the same as yesterday; mouth a little sticky, not so bitter. No stool; frequent and copious discharges of urine; icterus of a lighter color; no anxiety; cough much less frequent; sputa clear, ropy, without any abnormal color.

In the night the patient had to be changed three times; bled a little from the nose.

Dulness of sound in the super- and sub-spinal regions of the right side. Sound clear at the base.

Crepitation in the super- and sub-spinal spaces, larger and moister than the previous day. The bellows'-murmur is less intense; the voice is not so shrill.

Same treatment.

Oct. 22.—Pulse normal; skin natural; thirst moderate; tongue natural; mouth without bitterness; appetite; no stool; urine not very copious; scarcely any headache; no icterus; no anxiety; no stitch in the side, except during a deep inspiration; cough pretty frequent; expectoration easy, not copious, only a little ropy phlegm. No sweat.

Dulness of sound a little less in the super- and sub-spinal regions; crepitans redux; bellows'-murmur still heard in these regions.—*Bryonia* 24 in solution.

Oct. 23.—Feels quite well, generally as well as locally.

A little dulness in the super- and sub-spinal regions. Respiration in the super-spinal region harsh, but without any rattle. In the sub-spinal fossa, the respiration is normal, but a little harsh; during a paroxysm of cough a few large vesicles are still heard to crepitate.

Treatment discontinued. Broths.

On the subsequent days, the strength returned, and the convalescence took place without any untoward symptom; the patient was discharged cured on the 6th of Nov. 1848.

CASE 29.—*Pneumonia of the left side, second stage.*

Oct. 25th, 1848, Billon, 16 years old, paper-hanger, was admitted in the ward St. Charles No. 6; the patient is of middling constitution, has never been subject to ganglionic engorgements, nor to any derangements that generally point to a scrofulous taint.

He is not subject to cough; except that, three months ago, he went to the hospital St. Antoine, where he remained a whole month under treatment for a cold. His cough was frequent, distressing, and sometimes accompanied by vomiting. No stitch in the side, but a tearing pain along the sternum. He did not expectorate; according to the statement of the patient, the breathing was just as oppressed then as it is to-day. He was bled once.

He had not felt any of this illness for some time, when he was suddenly taken ill last Saturday. The day previous he felt well; he had done several errands, without feeling any unpleasant symptoms; he was in the habit of walking barefooted, but he does not recollect having taken cold previous to his illness. He did not cough any.

Saturday morning, on rising, he felt well as usual, ate his breakfast, and went to his work. Three or four hours after this, he was taken with a stitch in the side and a dry and distressing cough. He had neither headache nor precursory chill. He continued his work all day, and ate his meals with a pretty good appetite. In the evening the stitch and the cough had grown worse. He had no chill. The cough was dry. Had a pretty quiet sleep.

Sunday morning he was about the same as Saturday evening; the stitch and the cough continued. He went to church, and then staid home all day. The stitch grew worse during the walk; the appetite was less; night pretty good.

Monday morning he attempted to go to his work, but at eight o'clock he had to lie down again. He felt on acute pain in the left side of the chest, cough, violent oppression, heat, intense thirst, and complete loss of appetite. No expectoration, no chill.

Tuesday, same symptoms. Same nausea and vomiting.

Oct. 25.—Came to the hospital, and showed the following symptoms:

No headache, no buzzing in the ears or dizziness. Face red, moist; eyes sparkling; striking depression of strength and spirits. Lies on his back. The patient remains in the position in which he is placed. When sitting up, he experiences a violent oppression; his countenance is expressive of suffering, and his speech is broken and distresses him.

Skin burning hot and dry.

Respiration frequent, labored; violent oppression; anxiety; pain towards the seventh, eight and ninth left intercostal spaces, in the middle thereof; the pain is somewhat aggravated by pressure, but more particularly by cough and a deep inspiration.

36 inspirations in a minute.

Cough frequent, dry, distressing. No expectoration.

Auscultation reveals dulness of sound in the lower half of the left lung posteriorly.

Bronchial murmur from the lower portion of the subspinal fossa to the base of the lung, heard only during an inspiration. During a deep inspiration a crepitation of small, dry vesicles is heard on the sides of the space where the bronchial murmur is located.

Loud resonance of the voice to the ear, marked bronchophony.

In the axilla, bronchial murmur is likewise heard, also a crepitant rattle.

On the right side and behind, the natural inspirations are rather strong.

In front, neither murmur nor rattle is heard on the left side.

No dulness of sound.

Pulse large, regular, resisting. Striking sounds of the heart.

Pulse 96.

The tongue and gums are covered with whitish pellicles; the velum is free from them. Anorexia, intense thirst.

No nausea, nor vomiting. Abdomen a little distended, painful; no stool since yesterday.

No treatment. Water and sugar.

Previous to his admission in the hospital, ten leeches had been applied to him.

Oct. 26.—Same as yesterday. Face red and burning; skin burning and dry. No sleep. Intense dyspnœa. Speech labored.

Stethoscopic signs the same as yesterday. The bronchophony is more marked; loud resonance of the voice.

Spit up a watery, vesicular mucus three or four times, without any streaks of blood.

Pulse 92, inspirations 36.

No treatment. Dr. Valleix hands him over to Dr. Tessier.—He was ordered two pitcherfuls of water and sugar; *Bryonia* 12, in solution, and also *Bryonia* 24, another solution. Diet.

At 6 in the evening, same as in the morning. Pulse the same. General and local symptoms the same.

At 9 o'clock, another paroxysm of fever, a little delirium; he gets up. Considerable oppression.

Pulse 116.—This condition continues until midnight.

Oct. 27.—After midnight, the patient had two liquid

stools, one copious, the other less so, he discharged some urine twice, which was not examined. Very little sweat, which continued in the forenoon. Pulse 92, respirations 36.

Skin burning and slightly moist; anxiety as yesterday; the stitch in the side is less acute. Dyspnœa less than last evening at 9, but about the same as in the day-time. No expectoration. Same treatment and diet.

In the evening, the patient is about the same as in the morning. The general symptoms are not much less intense. The bronchial murmur has shifted to the middle of the sub-spinal fossa; it has almost disappeared low down, where a few vesicles are heard to crepitate during the ordinary inspirations. Where the bellows'-murmur terminates, crepitation is heard during the cough and during a deep inspiration.

Pulse 84 to 88; 36 inspirations.

Oct. 28.—Slight sweat in the night, sound sleep. Feels much better to-day. The general symptoms have ceased almost entirely; the patient's countenance is almost natural; the previous depression has disappeared, and has given place to a feeling of ease; the patient sits up in bed, and says he feels well. Pulse down to 56. Skin warm, like the breath; no oppression; a little cough without expectoration.

The bronchial murmur is limited to the space previously indicated; all around one hears, like yesterday, the crepitation of moist, large, unequal vesicles.

Pulse 56, inspirations 32.—Two solutions of *Bryonia;* water and sugar. Diet. In the evening, same symptoms. Pulse 44.

Oct. 29.—The improvement continues; the dulness decreases.

Pulse 44; inspirations 28.

Same treatment. Broths.

In the evening, same pulse; moisture.

Oct. 30.—Pulse regular, 40; inspirations 24.

Countenance cheerful; the patient had eaten his broth with an appetite.

Cough not frequent, easy, dry. No sweat in the night; no stool; the urine no more copious than natural; a little thirst and appetite; skin dry, mildly warm. Complete disappearance of the dulness; bellow's-murmur and crepitation during the ordinary inspirations have disappeared; but, when coughing or drawing a deep breath, the crackling of large moist vesicles is heard, especially in the sub-spinal fossa; it is less abundant in the lower portion of the chest. The respiration is rather harsh on a level with the spine of the scapula. Here the voice has as yet a more powerful resonance than on the right side.

Feeling of ease, no anxiety. Good sleep; stool regular.

Same treatment; broths and soups.

Nov. 1st.—Same symptoms.—Two pitcherfuls of water and sugar; *Bryonia* 12, in solution, one spoonful only; broths and soups.

Nov. 2 and 3.—Same treatment and regimen.

Nov. 4.—Two allowances; no medicine.

Nov. 5.—Same treatment; a little dry cough, but very seldom; the patient gets stronger every day; keen appetite. Pulse regular, 56.

Nov. 6.—A little bronchophony about a quarter of an inch from the spine of the scapula. No rattle. Pulse 48; inspirations 20.

This case, which has been related with the greatest care by Dr. Duhamel, attending physician under my respected colleague Dr. Valleix, offers a very peculiar interest. The patient was transferred to me by Dr. Valleix at the request of his pupils, who considered this case a fair criterium of the efficacy of homœopathic treatment.

I am aware that no serious conviction can be based upon an isolated case. But in this instance the cases which preceded, and those that will follow it, render such evidence as the above case involves, unimpeachable.

CASE 30.—*Pneumonia of the right lung.*

Lambert César, aged 60 years, carpenter, of a nervous temperament and a good constitution, and who had never been seriously sick, was, about a month previous to his admission in the hospital, attacked with a paroxysm during which he lost his senses, and for which he was bled at the arm. This paroxysm did not leave any disagreeable consequences behind, except an acute supra-orbital neuralgia which frequently disturbed his sleep. Since the events of February this man had undergone violent exertions and many privations. In the midst of these debilitating circumstances he was attacked with dysentery for which he was treated at the hospital Sainte-Marguérite, ward Sainte-Cécile No. 18, for about a fortnight, to date from Oct. 5th, 1848. On th 18th of Nov. he was fully convalescent, when he descended into the yard to wash his hands and face; on this day the weather was colder than usual; while he was washing himself, he did not feel any unpleasant symptom; but at breakfast, an hour or two after the washing, he felt ill and lost his appetite; soon after a violent chill ran over him, an intense heat broke out about his head, thence spread all over his body, giving rise to prickings and uneasiness in the extremities. Soon after he was taken with a violent headache and an acute stitch in the side, which deprived him of sleep. In the night an obstinate cough with bloody sputa, and an intense thirst, tormented him with the other distresses. Next morning these symptoms remained about the same with an equal intensity and without any other change supervening.

Nov. 20th the following symptoms were noticed: face red and animated; eye lively; the patient lies on his back, slightly turned to the left side; in other respects neither prostration nor nervousness. Pulse 120; cough frequent, dry, in paroxysms, hacking; expectoration copious, resembling in color the juice of prunes, a little blood-streaked, rather tough, adhering to the vessel like liquid glue; headache pretty acute; had to be changed once last night on account of the sweat. Tongue looks natural. No nausea; no vomiting. Had not had any stool for two or three days past; urine less copious than usual; the stitch is located opposite the right breast; not much anxiety.

Percussion yields a dull sound over the whole of the right chest, posteriorly; in front the sound is normal; nothing remarkable on the left side.

Auscultation reveals an intense bellows'-murmur over the whole surface of the right chest, posteriorly; but the point where it is most intense is opposite the spine of the scapula; here a very fine crepitation was heard, but only during the cough.—*Bryonia* 12 and 24, two solutions.

Nov. 21.—Pulse 112; skin rather moist, a little warmer than naturally; cough less frequent, sputa partially bloody; of a reddish-brown color, and partially of a green color like a marmelade of green prunes; the sputa is viscid, not vesicular; the stitch, as painful as yesterday, has shifted to the edge of the false ribs; sleepless night, with headache, and very restless. Tongue covered with a whitish coating, without any redness at the borders; thirst intense; no nausea; no vomiting.

The supra-spinal fossa yields a good sound; the sound in the sub-spinal fossa is rather dull; at the base of the chest the sound is incomplete.

Auscultation reveals the following signs: No rattle, no bellows'-murmur in the supra-spinal fossa. Bellows-murmur and crepitant rattle in the sub-spinal fossa.

5

At the base, the bellows-'murmur is less intense than in the last-named space; sub-crepitant rattle.

The celebral functions seem slightly irritated; his speech is short, his *movements sudden and quick*, but his mind perfectly clear.

No change of treatment.

Nov. 22.—Pulse 112, hard and full; copious perspiration all night, quiet and a little sleep; skin moist, heat normal; face rather animated, celebral excitement the same, the patient seems even a little flighty; the supra-orbital neuralgia is very distressing, which might perhaps account for his restlessness and delirious irritation. Cough not very frequent, sputa remains the same as regards color and quantity, except that some of it assumes a yellow-brown color, and becomes blood-streaked and bloody; tongue natural, thirst not very great.

Marked dulness from the spine of the scapula to the lower angle of this bone; from this point to the base of the thorax it gradually disappears.

Loud bellows'-murmur in the sub-spinal fossa, especially during an expiration; fine and very even, vesicular crepitation in the same region. The murmur grows fainter in proportion as one approaches the base of the thorax, but in the neighborhood of the vertebral column, from the base of the chest to the spine of the scapula, the crepitation is unequal.

The stitch in the side is less acute, the patient is able to blow his nose, and to cough without much trouble.

Same treatment.

Nov. 23.—Pulse 112; face less red and the countenance less animated; the skin remains covered with a slight moisture; tongue coated white, thirst intense, stitch much less. The neuralgia remains very acute; the patient had a stool this morning. Cough not very frequent; the expectoration as copious as on the previous days; but the greenish color of the sputa is lighter, and some of the expectoration is of a pale yellow color; it is equally adhering and tough.

Dulness in the sub-spinal fossa, decreasing towards the base of the thorax; during an expiration a bellows-murmur is heard in the sub-spinal fossa; but less intense than on the preceding days; likewise a crepitant rattle; a sub-crepitant rattle is heard toward the base, especially in the neighborhood of the spinal column.

Same treatment.

Nov. 24—Pulse 92; cough less intense; the sputa contains large air-vesicles; it is of a lighter color than before, preserving however the greenish and pinkish tinge; a copious sweat broke out last night; this morning the temperature is about natural. The stitch extends across the forepart of the chest, and is not very acute. Tongue slightly coated white, moist; thirst moderate; the patient had a scanty stool last night.

Slight dulness in the sub-spinal fossa; at the base of the chest the sound is slightly obscured.

Bellows'-murmur and crepitation in the sub-spinal fossa; sub-crepitant rattle at the base.

Much less restless than previously; towards evening, the patient again became drenched with sweat, which had a marked acid smell.—*Bryonia* 12.

Nov. 25.—Pulse 104; cough slight and not frequent; sputa partly tough, partly vesicular; their greenish tinge is growing lighter; some of it continues blood-streaked and of a pink color, and strongly adhering; it is much less profuse.

The patient has lost his cerebral irritation, and now feels rather weak in the limbs; has had a good night; the tongue is a little red; feels somewhat thirsty, and the skin is rather hot; the stitch has left him.

Dulness of sound in the sub-spinal fossa; otherwise the sounds are normal all over the chest.

Loud bellows'-murmur in the region of the bronchial roots, crepitation in the sub-spinal fossa, sub-crepitant rattle towards the base.—*Bryonia* 24.

Nov. 26.—Pulse 80, hard and full; perspired a good deal last night; herpes labialis on both lips; tongue coated whitish; not much thirst; cough rare; the expectoration is of a lighter color and not very copious. Had a good night.

Neither dulness, nor bellows'-murmur any where in the chest; in the sub-spinal fossa, especially towards the vertebral column, a sub-crepitant rattle with unequal humid vesicles is heard.

Nov. 27.—No marked change in the condition of the patient.

Nov. 28.—Pulse 80; skin naturally warm; a little cough; the sputa is greenish, scanty, and resembles nasal mucus in color and consistence; the appetite reappears;—broth.

In the sub-spinal fossa the sound is slightly obscure; respiration a little harsh, with a few vesicles of crepitant and mucous rattle.

Nov. 29.—Pulse 80; sputa of a light-yellow color; no cough; some dulness of sound interiorly to the scapular spine, with a little bellows'-murmur during an expiration; no rattle.—Broths and soups.

Nov. 30.—Pulse 76; sputa of a lemon-color, vesicular, ropy, not very copious; slight obscurity of sound interiorly to the spine of the scapula; a little bellows'-murmur during an expiration.

During the following days the resolution takes place. The patient leaves the hospital on the 11th of January, 1849, after having completely restored her strength.

CASE 31.—*Pneumonia of the right side.*

Wach, aged 33 years, tailor, was admitted Dec. 9th, 1848, ward St. Benjamin, No. 27.

Was taken sick on the 3d. First he was taken with

a violent pain in the right side, chill, and intense headache; frequent paroxysms of cough distressed him; he raised something, but did not see any blood until the 7th. Lost his appetite from the commencement of his illness. Applied three times for admission in some hospital, and had to wait until the 9th, during which time his disease kept growing worse. On the day of his admission, he showed the following symptoms:

Constitution pretty sound; skin warm and covered with sweat; if he sits up in bed or talks, he trembles a good deal; breathing hurried; complains of an acute pain in the right side, which he has had from the commencement of the attack. Percussion yields a marked dulness in the middle third of the percussed lung. Auscultation reveals a loud bellows'-murmur; the sputa is opaque, bloody, adhering to the sides of the vessel; pulse 104. Tongue coated; the patient complains of a bitter taste in the mouth; he has no appetite, but a good deal of thirst; has no pain in the bowels, and goes to stool regularly; head heavy and painful; face pale, livid; the symptoms show that there is serious danger of suppuration. Before coming to the hospital, he had contented himself with drinking Linden-tea. In the evening he was ordered two pitcherfuls of water and sugar, and two solutions of *Bryonia*, one 12, the other 24; strict diet.

Dec. 11.—The patient is found in nearly the same position; he does not feel less pain; the bellows'-murmur is a little worse, heard over the three upper fourths of the lung; pulse 108; *Bryonia* 12, two solutions.

Dec. 12.—Pulse 104; no improvement; the murmur continues; sputa bloody. Same treatment. In the evening the patient feels better, and raises more easily.

Dec. 13.—Pulse 96; upon the whole, the patient feels much better than before; sputa less red, the murmur is much less; it is only heard in the upper half of the chest. In the lower half, a sub-crepitant rattle is heard. Countenance looks better.

Bryonia and *Sulphur* 12 in solution, alternately.

From 11 o'clock in the forenoon until 3 in the afternoon, the patient suffered a good deal of pain in the side, with much difficulty of breathing.

Dec. 14.—The patient is much better; he is quieter; the skin continues warm and moist. Pulse 72; sputa no longer blood-streaked. The patient had some refreshing sleep; a faint bellows'-murmur continues to be heard in the sub-spinal fossa.—*Bryonia* in solution.

Dec. 15.—No sleep last night; no pain, pulse 64. No oppression; he only shows a little bellows'-murmur and sub-crepitant rattle on a level with the spine of the scapula. The sputa is mucous and vesicular. Continue *Bryonia.*

Dec. 16.—Sputa continues viscid. The murmur has disappeared, only a sub-crepitant rattle remains on a level with the spine of the scapula. The patient had some sleep, feels better; the skin is warm and moist; pulse 68. *Bryonia* and *Phosphorus* in solution, alternately.

Dec. 17.—Only a little sub-crepitant rattle high up. *Phosphorus* in solution.

Dec. 18.—Respiration perfect in the whole extent of the lungs; pulse 60; the skin continues a little warm; the patient has an appetite. *Bryonia;* broth.

Dec. 19.—The patient feels very well; is still unable to draw a long breath.—Broths, soups, and *Phosphorus*, three spoonfuls a day, until Dec. 25.—Respiration perfect; the patient eats a little piece of chicken.

Dec. 29.—Two meals; his strength returns very speedily; he remains in the ward as a laborer until January 29th, 1849.

CASE 32.—*Pneumonia of the right side.*

Ward Sainte-Anne, No. 7. Doré, 72 years old, a day-servant, admitted Dec. 30th, 1848.

Dec. 24, the patient was attacked with a violent chill, which lasted two hours; she felt a painful stitch in the right side, opposite the breast. Soon after a hot fever set in, with cough, and an expectoration that was not very clearly described by the patient.

This woman had been in a room without fire during the extremely cold weather of this season; she remained in her room until the 7th day, without any attendance. Had enjoyed good health previously; in spite of her advanced age, this woman had retained a certain degree of vigor.

Dec. 31.—Dulness of sound in the whole right side of the chest; bellows'-murmur in the same region. Painful stitch in the side, dyspnœa, fever, cough, bloody sputa.—*Bryonia* 12, in the day-time; *Bryonia* 24 at night.

January 1st, 1849.—General expression of debility; dyspnœa; short, frequent, sobbing respiration; flushes at the malar region, tongue coated blackish, thick, dry; eyes full of gum. Intense fever, pulse 92, small. Yellowish lumpy sputa, with a few streaks of blood. Acute pain around the right breast. No sleep.

Dulness in the whole right side; auscultation does reveal any signs; the lung does not perform the act of respiration; only bronchophonic resonance is heard when the patient talks.—*Bryonia*, two solutions.

Jan. 2.—Increased prostration; the patient lies on her back. Respiration short and slow; speech short and broken; skin warm; pulse feeble, 92; tongue dry; fuliginous; acute pains in the side. No sleep.

Stethoscopic signs the same, except a few crepitating vesicles here and there; in the other parts of the lung, a marked bellows'-sound. Not much expectoration; lumpy, thick sputa, without blood.—*Bryonia* 12; *Phosphorus* 12, alternately.

Jan. 3.—General appearance improved; breathing a

little fuller; the tongue became moist; is less coated. Slept three hours last night. Pulse up to 100, fuller. The skin is cooler and moister; the stitch is still very painful; less prostration; the patient commences to stir about.

A stool; stethoscopic signs the same.

The patient complains of pains at the sacrum; two large red patches are discovered at this place, one of which exhibits two dry black sloughs.—Two broths. Bryonia 12, *Phosphorus* 12 in solution, alternately.

Jan. 4.—General condition much better; had a good sleep last night. The patient feels much more comfortable, raises herself in bed with a certain vigor, talks and jests. The breathing is less frequent and deeper; the cough is less; sputa thinner, rather frothy, in short fragments, blood-streaked. The stitch is not so constant, and is scarcely felt, except during the cough; skin of the temperature of the breath; pulse 86.

Crepitans redux at the summit of the lung.—Two thin soups.—*Bryonia* 24 and *Phosphorus* 12 alternately.

Jan. 5.—Sputa in flakes, thinner, frothy, vesicular: pulse 80; increase of strength.—Continue the medicine.

Jan. 6.—Feels stronger; had some sleep. Skin cool; pulse 80, tongue moist; appetite; cough less frequent, sputa vesicular; the respiratory murmur is heard in the whole right side of the chest, but less distinctly than in the opposite side. The resonance is restored; the pain is only felt when coughing, and is then much less than before; general appearance very good; the two scabs on the sacrum fall off, the redness is less. The patient lies alternately on her back and on the side. Two light soups, milk.—*Bryonia* and *Phosphorus* alternately.

Jan. 7.—Gradual improvement; the patient begs for food.—Same treatment.

Jan. 8.—Long paroxysm of cough in the night; the

patient says she never had a catarrh previous to this sickness.—*Bryonia* and *Ipecac.* in solution alternately.

Jan. 9.—Pulse 84; cough in the night.—*Bryonia* and *Belladonna* in solution, alternately.

Jan. 10.—Skin cool, pulse down to 76; increase of strength, better appetite; cough less frequent; easy expectoration; the respiratory murmur becomes stronger; no abnormal sounds.—*Bryonia* in solution, two spoonfuls; Belladonna in solution.

Jan. 11.—Two small ulcers remain in the places where the scabs have sloughed off; the rednesses have disappeared from the sacrum.—*Ipec.* in solution.

Jan. 12 to 20.—No medicine was given; every now and then the patient had an attack of cough in the night; she went on improving, however, and recovered her strength. On the 20th, all the stethoscopic signs had ceased; the cough gave place to a clear, vesicular expectoration. The convalescence took place with extreme ease. The patient was permitted to remain in the ward for some time as an act of favor.

This case shows that one ought not to despair too readily. This pneumonia, which had been so long neglected, had not yet passed into the stage of suppuration when we commenced the treatment. Hence the conclusion was that the patient might still be cured, and she was cured with a surprising promptitude.

CASE 33.—*Pneumonia of the left side.*

Rouel, 70 years old, carpenter, was admitted in the ward St. Benjamin, No. 8, Jan. 29th, 1848.

Had a pretty good constitution. Twelve years ago he had an attack of pulmonary catarrh, which he describes pretty accurately. The left lung was affected. At the age of 30, this lung had likewise been inflamed. Nothing else of consequence to be related concerning the former life of this patient.

He had never had a cold before; but this year he had

been more exposed, and took a cold which he kept for about two months, when, in the night of the 24th of January, he was suddenly taken with a chill followed by fever. At the same time he felt a pain which first shifted about in the chest, and finally localized itself near the left nipple, where it became very acute. The cough which had not been very frequent until then, and gave rise to a mucous expectoration, increased, and became painful and distressing. Headache, fever. Five days previous, the patient experienced a feeling of sickness, which he described as a sense of weariness and lameness; nevertheless he had worked all day in his shop on the 23d.

Jan. 29.—Considerable dyspnœa; respiration frequent; speech broken; acute pain in the side which caused a distortion of the features at every inspiration. This pain was seated opposite the left nipple, and is aggravated by percussion. Cheeks flushed, violent headache; hot skin and frequent pulse; frequent cough; viscid, adhering sputa, of a bright pale-yellow color; some of the expectoration contains a little blood which is, however, well mixed up with it. No appetite, dry tongue, coated a thick yellowish fur; stool natural.

Auscultation of the left side reveals a loud bellows'-murmur, specially on starting from the lower angle of the sternum; resonance of the voice; above, starting from the superior half of the scapula, a few crepitating vesicles. Dulness of sound over the whole lower half. On the right side the sounds are normal; respiration without any abnormal murmurs, but weaker than in a state of health; the chest does not dilate fully; the pain prevents a full dilatation.—*Bryonia* 12 and 24, two solutions.

Jan. 30.—This morning, a quantity of sputa of the color of barley-sugar, viscid, the lower part strongly adhering to the vessel; the other portion the more tenacious the greater the quantity. Fever, hot skin, pulse 100; same symptoms, same physical signs.

Evening:—The patient has coughed less than before, feels a little better, has had several short naps. Skin covered with perspiration, the shirt is wet. A stool. No other change.—*Bryonia* 12 and *Phosphorus* 12 in solution, alternately.

Jan. 31.—Profuse sweat all night; the patient had to be changed once. Sleep, less cough, viscid sputa of the color of barley-sugar. In the morning, cool skin, pulse 64, regular, soft; inspirations deeper and easier. The stitch in the side is much less; is only felt during the cough and on percussing the chest, whereas it was constantly felt previously. The headache is less; the patient feels better; the general appearance is very satisfactory, tongue moist. No stool.

The physical signs are the same, except that the breathing is fuller, and that on the left side the bellows'-murmur, and on the right side a normal respiration are more distinct.—Continue *Bryonia* and *Phosphorus*.

Feb. 1st.—Last night the cough was more frequent than the day previous; three or four times the patient raised rusty sputa; at other times phlegm. Pulse 60, warmth like that of the breath, respiration deeper. The headache is much less; the pain in the side is slight, and is only felt during the violent paroxysms of cough. The tongue continues a little dry, the appetite returns. No more sweat.

The dulness of sound is gone; a little more bellows'-murmur on the left, low down. Respiration feeble, without any abnormal murmurs.—*Bryonia* 24.

Feb. 2.—General condition pretty fair; tongue moist, face natural; the flush is gone, respiration almost normal; pain in the side very slight. Pulse 60; raises only mucus.

Inspiration a little harsher than on the sound side, but expansive and general.

Appetite.—Broth. *Bryonia* 24.

Feb. 3.—Inspiration increases in volume; same signs as above. Pulse 60. General condition good. Broths, soups.—Bryonia only a few spoonfuls.

Feb. 4.—Full convalescence.

Now and then a few turns of cough, and a few dull pains shifting from one part of the thorax to the other, and from the shoulder to the thorax; but they do not trouble the patient. In a few days the breathing became as full on the left as on the right side; no abnormal murmur in the whole extent of the chest.

Feb. 24.—The patient expects to be discharged from day to day. Leaves March 13th, 1848.

CASE 34.—*Pneumonia of the right side.*

A young man of 25 years, whose name has been forgotten, was admitted on the 24th of April, 1849, ward St. Benjamin, No. 31.

April 20th, about 4 o'clock in the evening, without any assignable cause, without any precursory symptoms, he was taken with a feeling of sickness; he left his work, went home, felt chilly; soon after a fever set in, with a stitch in the right antero-lateral portion of the thorax. In the night the breathing became more difficult, more hurried; sweat broke out. He remained without any medical treatment until the evening of 24th of April.

We found the following symptoms: Face flushed, expressive of suffering. Respiration frequent, not very full. Tongue flat, moist, covered with a thin whitish coating. Cough loose, not very frequent; raised some viscid coherent sputa, strongly adhering to the vessel, of a beautiful apricot-color, and mixed here and there with fine streaks of blood. Acute fever; skin hot, equally covered with sweat all over; pulse frequent, large, soft, 120. Frontal headache; loss of appetite, intense thirst. Has not had any passage from the bowels for two days; only one stool since the commencement of his sickness.

Percussion yields dulness of sound in the upper portion of the right lung; the left side yields a good sound.

Auscultation discloses a bellows'-murmur in the whole extent of the right lung, without rattle; on the left side the respiration is normal, only not so full as in a state of health; the inspirations are frequent and not very deep; the lung is only imperfectly dilated. Painful stitch below the right nipple, preventing the expansion of the chest.—*Bryonia* 12, in solution.

April 25.—Same symptoms in the morning; profuse sweat, hot skin, pulse frequent, 118, 120.—*Bryonia* 12.

April 26.—Same sweat, affording no relief. Had no sleep.

Frontal headache; flushed face, tongue moist, flat, coated white; thirst intense.

Respiration frequent; stitch not so painful. Same physical signs, except that the respiration is a little deeper; the bellows'-murmur in the whole right lung is more distinct; it might be considered typical of this class of signs. On the left side the vesicular murmur is heard more plainly. The expectoration is not excessive, but extremely characteristic. Pulse 115. No stool.—*Bryonia* 12 and *Phosphorus* 12 in solution, alternately.

April 27.—Skin moist, sweat less copious. Pulse 115. Cough not very frequent; sputa less colored. No headache.

In the night, painful exacerbation of the stitch in the side; for two hours, pain in the whole of the right side, as far as the shoulder; anxiety. No pain this morning.

Same physical signs.— Same treatment.

In the evening a few crepitating vesicles at the right middle portion. Pulse 108.

April 28.—Perceptible improvement; breathing easier;

cough not frequent, expectoration almost free from blood, but continues viscid. The stitch is only painful during the cough and when drawing a long breath. No headache. Tongue moist, and a little coated; thirst less. Skin moist, heat milder; pulse 104. The patient feels well, slept some.

Crepitans redux at the middle portion of the lung. No stool.—Same treatment.

April 29.—Skin gently warm, pulse down to 62. No stitch; cough rare; raises only phlegm.

During a turn of cough, auscultation discloses crepitation in the whole extent of the lung; some bellows'-murmur in the sub-spinal region, near the axillary border of the scapula.—*Bryonia* 24.

April 30.—Temperature of the skin and pulse the same.—Confluent miliaria on the chest, abdomen, forehead.

Cough rare; raises a little mucus. No stitch in the side. Resonance; a few crepitating vesicles here and there. No bellows'-murmur.

Slight stomatitis; tongue thickly coated yellowish, with red edges; gums with a whitish border around the teeth.—Broth. *Bryonia* in solution.

May 2.—The miliaria is disappearing. Skin cool; pulse 62. Stomatitis.

Cough very trifling, not painful, no expectoration.

The respiration on the affected side is a little harsher than in health; no abnormal noises.

No stool. Appetite.—Broth, soups. *Bryonia.*

May 3.—The eruption is gone. Complete convalescence. An allowance. Discharged May 10th.

CASE 35.—*Pneumonia of the right side.*

Delormey, a man of 59 years, small stature, worn-out and thin constitution, admitted July 10th, ward St. Benjamin, No. 5.

July 5th he was taken with illness in the evening; he

threw up his dinner, went to bed; he felt chilly, fever set in, and afterwards an acute pain near the right nipple. The patient begins to cough, and next morning he raises a viscid, rusty substance. No treatment; only quiet in bed.

July 10th, the day of his admission, the patient presented the following condition: Flushed and animated face, rather thin; tongue moist and lined with a thick yellowish-white coating; thirst, loss of appetite, constipation.

Skin hot and dry; pulse soft, large, 95. Respiration frequent, short, hurried; speech broken, exciting the cough; the cough is frequent, in short paroxysms, giving rise to a scanty expectoration of small quantities, viscid, blood-streaked phlegm. The stitch under the right nipple is very painful, aggravated by cough; while coughing the patient holds this part with his hands.

Percussion yields a complete dulness of sound in the lower half of the thorax; in the upper portion the resonance is good. Above the spine of the scapula a few crepitating vesicles are heard, and above it a loud bellows'-murmur, especially during an inspiration; bronchophony. Above the spine, frequent crepitations in the whole summit of the lung.—*Bryonia* 12 in solution; water and sugar.

July 11.—Same symptoms; pulse 100.—*Bryonia* 12 and 24, two solutions.

July 12.—General condition the same. Warm skin, pulse 95. Dyspnœa the same; frequent cough; expectoration scanty, but characteristic. The stitch in the side is a little less, painful only during the cough. In the lower portion of the lung the crepitation is more frequent; but in the lower portion a loud bellows'-murmur continues to be heard. Dulness of sound. Resolution has commenced low down. High up the bellows'-murmur is pretty loud, with a few crepitating vesicles during the cough.

The patient coughed a good deal in the night; slept only a few moments. Constipation. *Bryonia* in solution 12, and 24, as above.

July 13.—Less fever; the skin is softer, pulse 75. The breathing is easier; the stitch is only felt during the cough; the patient raises a little viscid, bloody matter.

Crepitation more frequent low down; the bellows'-murmur is only distinctly heard above the spine of the shoulder-blade.—*Bryonia* and *Phosphorus* in solution, alternately.

July 14.—Same symptoms. A stool during the day. Tongue coated the same. Same treatment.

July 15.—Skin soft and a little moist; face less flushed; no headache; the patient has grown thinner; pulse 70.

Breathing easier; cough less frequent; a little characteristic sputa. The stitch has almost ceased. The patient feels better; had a few naps in the night. Tongue coated; thirst moderate; no appetite. A passage.

Resolution is fully going on in the lower portion of the lung; crepitation prevails in this part; slight bellows'-murmur during an expiration, and here and there very distinct. In the upper portion dulness of sound, loud murmur.—Same treatment.

July 17.—Skin warm, pulse 65. Dyspnœa; cough rare, scarcely any expectoration; expectoration more mucous, less viscid, more scattering; a few streaks of blood. The patient slept some last night. Tongue still coated. Same appetite.

Same physical signs. Same treatment. Broth.

July 22.—General condition good; no fever; pulse 60. In the evening, a little exacerbation. The patient feels well, the breathing is not hurried but not so full as in health. The stitch has disappeared. Cough rare; raises scarcely any mucus.

Tongue continues thickly coated; the secretions are restored. Same appetite.

The resolution has been somewhat wavering, and has not taken place with the some regularity as in other cases. In the lower portion, crepitation prevails; all this time only a bellows'-murmur was heard; now the crepitant rattle is more frequent and more distinct; a little murmur is heard here and there.

July 30.—Convalescent. The patient eats well and leaves his bed; the cough has ceased; the chest dilates perfectly. He is kept in the ward on account of his poverty, but he is a very troublesome and refractory inmate. He eats every-thing that he can lay hold of, and has several attacks of indigestion. Every morning, early, he goes down in the yard to smoke his pipe.

August 15th, he was attacked with erysipelas of the nose and an acute inflammation of the nostrils, which were filled with dry crusts. In spite of this attack, and contrary to all our warnings, he continues to go down in the morning and smoke. On the third day the nose became red, and the tip livid; a double bronchitis sets in, with difficult catarrhal expectoration, mucous rattle on both sides of the chest, extreme oppression, acute fever, prostration, delirium, aphonia. These symptoms continue to grow worse; marasmus sets in; Aug. 22d coma, and death on the 24th.

Post-mortem examination: The bronchia were completely obstructed with a thick mucus; the mucous membrane was red and injected; no pneumonia.

The parenchyma of the right lung, which had been inflamed, was perfectly sound and crepitating, there were a few very fine cellular adhesions between the two pleuræ.

CASE 36.—*Pneumonia.*

Gruel, a woman of 27 years old, having a good constitution, of good health generally, regular menstruation, was taken sick July 10th.

For two days past, she had not felt well, had no appetite, felt tired, had a little diarrhœa, but continued her work. On the 10th, towards evening, she felt worse, had a chill, fever, headache, and from time to time an acute pain under the right breast; cough set in. Kept her bed for four days without any treatment.

July 14, she showed the following symptoms: flushed face, frontal headache, tongue moist with a thin white coating; intense thirst, loss of appetite; watery sweat with great heat, pulse soft and large, 95.

Respiration hurried, high up, constantly interrupted by frequent and distressing paroxysms of cough; profuse viscid, rusty sputa, of the color of barley-sugar, over which floats a mucous, vesicular, frothy liquid; acute pain under the right breast, aggravated by the cough.

Since her sickness, the patient has had two diarrhœic stools every day.

No symptoms in the left side of the chest; in the right side we find: marked dulness in the whole upper part of the lung; expiratory murmur very distinct; bronchophony. Crepitating vesicles high up.—*Bryonia* 12 in solution.

July 15.—Same symptoms.—*Bryonia* 12 and 24 two solutions.

July 16.—Less headache; face less animated; skin warm, moist; pulse 90, same as above. The stitch is less constant, aggravated by the cough, which remains the same. The patient complains of the cough tiring her; she is unable to sleep; the characteristic sputa is much less; the expectoration consists almost entirely of the clear, frothy liquid.

Tongue moist, slightly coated white; one liquid stool in the twenty-four hours; no pain in the bowels; thirst moderate; no appetite.

Dulness of sound in the lower portion of the lung much less; the bellows'-murmur is intermingled with a large number of moist crepitating vesicles. The respiration is fuller, less frequent in the upper portion of the lung; loud bellows'-murmur below the scapular spine.—*Bryonia* 12 and *Phosphorus* 12 in alternation.

July 17.—General improvement, skin less hot, pulse 70; no headache; breathing not very quick, but the paroxysms of cough continue to fatigue the patient. The expectoration is only composed of a quantity of frothy liquid; the stitch is much less painful during the cough; tongue moist, scarcely coated; appetite; a liquid stool in the twenty-four hours.

The resolution is taking place very fully in the lower portion of the lung; the bellows'-murmur has ceased; the crepitation is more scattered almost over the whole upper portion of the lung; a little bellows'-murmur is still heard near the scapular spine, in the neighborhood of the axilla.—Continue *Bryonia* and *Phosphorus.*

July 19.—Skin of the temperature of the breath, face natural, no headache; pulse 60. General condition good; slept some last night. Cough continues frequent, distressing, with mucous, vesicular, clear expectoration; thirst natural; tongue good; appetite; another liquid stool.

The lower portion of the lung respires less freely than the sound lung, but without any abnormal murmur; crepitation in the upper portion; no bellows'-murmur. —Bryonia; broth, soup.

July 20.—Same condition; the stitch has returned, causing an acute pain near the breast; cough less, less long and distressing; mucous expectoration; less crepitation with smaller vesicles, in the upper portion of the lung.—*Arnica* in solution, soup.

July 22.—Complete disappearance of the crepitant rattle; convalescence.—Bryonia and diet as before.

July 24.—No trace of pneumonia, but long and frequent paroxysms of cough followed by a mucous, clear, abundant expectoration. This cough fatigues the patient; it breaks out again from the least cause, wakes her at night. The general condition, however, is good; no fever, no abnormal murmurs of any consequence. The appetite is good; the patient recovers her strength.

This cough continued the same until the beginning of August; it was removed by Belladonna and Aconite. —Discharged cured, Aug. 8th.

CASE 37.—*Pneumonia.*

Mallez, aged 36 years, admitted in the ward St. Benjamin, No. 35, August 21st, 1849.

In the month of June last, this patient had been treated in our hospital for a very severe attack of cholera; after which he resumed his work.

August 16th, he experienced without any assignable cause, a feeling of illness, anorexia, weariness; Aug. 17, he was taken with a chill, fever, acute pain in the left side, cough. Kept his bed until the 21st, without treatment.

We found the following symptoms: Face red, animated; breathing short and frequent; frontal headache; tongue moist and white-coated; intense thirst.

Skin hot and dry; pulse large, soft, 110. Painful stitch in the side, like neuralgia, located in the seventh intercostal space, with painful stitches in front and behind. The pain is so violent that the patient tries to suppress his cough. Breathing frequent and suppressed; cough comes by paroxysms. Moderate expectoration of viscid sputa of the color of barley-sugar.

Percussion yields a dull sound on the left side, in the lower portion of the thorax, from the spine to the shoulder blade. On the right side, the sound is normal.

On the left side, auscultation reveals a short bellows'-murmur during an expiration, rather distant from the ear and located in the larger bronchial tubes. No very distinct rattle high up; on the right side, the respiration is feeble; the chest dilates hardly.

Constipation; no pain any where else.—*Bryonia* 12 in solution.

Aug. 22.—Same symptoms in the morning; the patient has a good deal of fever, did not sleep any. Pulse 110.—Continue *Bryonia.*

Aug. 23.—Considerable improvement; skin softly warm; pulse 60. No headache, moist tongue, not much thirst. Stitch less painful; occasional dartings. Little cough; expectoration viscid, continues a little colored.

Inspiration feebler, quieter, full on the right side; on the left side, numerous crepitating vesicles in the lower and posterior portion of the lung; same bellows'-murmur. A passage.—*Bryonia* 24.

Aug. 24.—Same state; pulse 52; skin cool. Stitch still painful at times; has all the character of neuralgia. Cough rare; does not raise much; scattered crepitation in the left lung; no bellows'-murmur; vesicular respiration on the right side much fuller.—Continue *Bryonia.*

August 25.—Complete resolution; respiration less quiet and expansive on the left side; normal on the right side; skin cool, pulse 48. Intercostal neuralgia continues; appetite.—Broth. *Bryonia.*

Aug. 26.—Regular convalescence; pulse 48.

On the days following the neuralgia attacked him several times. On the first of September the patient took a walk which fatigued him; he had a fever all night, pulse 60.

Sept. 9—17.—The neuralgia has left him. Discharged cured.

CASE 38.—*Pneumonia of the left lung in front,* (a remarkable circumstance, so far as the cause and seat of the disease are concerned.)

Thirion, 43 years. Admitted Sept. 6th, 1849, ward St. Benjamin, No. 9.

Sept. 3d, the patient was employed in unloading a wagon; two men placed on his shoulder a bag when one of them let go of his hold, and the bag fell heavily upon Thirion's shoulder. At the same moment the patient experienced a severe pain in the front part of the chest, opposite the attachment of the pectoral muscles and the serratus major; nevertheless he carried his load to the third story, but was obliged to quit work. The whole of this and the following day, he felt a pain, malaise; he spit a little blood; he kept quiet without going to bed.

Sept. 5, in the morning, he was taken with a chill, followed by fever; he commenced to cough; next day he came to the hospital with the following symptoms:

Face red, bloated; respiration frequent, marked dyspnœa. Tongue moist, coated white; intense thirst; no appetite.

Skin warm; pulse large, soft, 115.

The pain was not confined to one spot like a stitch, but spread over a portion of the front part of the left lung. The pain is aggravated by the breathing and coughing.

Expectoration profuse, viscid, resembling a thick solution of gum, which is covered by a little characteristic blood-streaked, not yet properly mixed sputa.

Dulness of sound all over the left anterior thoracic region, and a portion of the lateral region. Every where else the sound is normal. Over the same space a loud and clear bellow's-murmur is heard, especially during an expiration; it hides in a great measure the sounds of the heart, which can only be perceived by an attentive ear and offer no abnormal sign. The murmur is heard in the whole of the axilla, and left side. Where the lateral and posterior portions unite, a crepitant rattle is heard; all over behind, vesicular respiration; no abnormal sign on the right side.—*Arnica* 6; *Phosphorus* 12, in alternation.

Sept. 7 and 8.—Same symptoms and physical signs. Pulse 115 to 120. Pain in the side, headache; cough frequent and painful; expectoration characteristic and profuse. No sleep; thirst, anorexia; constipation. Sept. 8 took *Bryonia*.

Sept. 9.—Headache; tongue dry, with whitish coating, red edges; slight stomatitis. Skin still hot, but rather moist; pulse large, soft, 106.

Breathing labored; dull pain, cough, profuse expectoration with sputa of the color of barley-sugar.

Same physical signs; a few vesicles are heard to crepitate here and there in the anterior middle portion of the left lung.—*Bryonia*.

Sept. 10.—No headache, tongue moister. Skin moist, not so hot; pulse 96. Cough less frequent; slept some last night; less rusty sputa. Pain in the side, or rather the lameness less.

Crepitans redux almost over the whole lung, with numerous vesicles; the sounds of the heart are more distinct than when they were disguised by the above-mentioned bellows'-murmur. A little appetite; a passage.—Diet. *Bryonia*.

Sept. 11.—Yesterday the patient who was rather contrary, exposed himself to a current of air. To day, the dyspnœa, fever and cough are worse; rusty sputa, viscid and copious. The bellows-murmur has reappeared in the whole forepart of the lung.—*Bryonia* and *Rhus-t.* 12, in alternation.

Sept. 12.—Considerable improvement. No headache. Tongue moist, scarcely coated. Skin moist; pulse 80. Cough rare, expectoration less and more mucous.

The secretions are restored.—*Bryonia* in solution.

Sept. 13.—No fever, pulse 60, skin cool; slept some last night. Cough and expectoration the same.

Crepitation of scattered vesicles. Appetite.—*Bryonia.*

Sept. 14.—Skin cool. Pulse 56. Raises some mucus; respiration normal. Appetite.—Broths. *Bryonia.*

Sept. 15.—Pulse 56. Complete convalescence. Appetite. Soups. No medicine.

Sept. 16.—Pulse the same. 17.—Pulse 48. 18.—Pulse 46.—An allowance. 19 and 20.—Pulse 46.—Discharged Oct. 10.

SECOND SERIES.

CASES OF PNEUMONIA THAT TERMINATED FATALLY.

CASE 39.—*Pneumonia.*

Roman, 43 years old, painter, was admitted on the 22d of March. Was of a feeble and nervous constitution, but had always enjoyed good health. Since the revolution of February, being without work and without means, he had to suffer all sorts of privations, even hunger; to gain a livelihood, he had to work at the embankments of the Champ de Mars. Smarting under the infliction of his moral sufferings much more than from his physical misery, he grew weaker from day to day, until March 17th, when he was attacked with a feeling of lameness in consequence of having been exposed to the rain all day. Next morning, he woke with a burning fever, a stitch in the side, and cough without expectoration. In this state he remained without any treatment from Saturday to Wednesday, on which day he was received at the hospital.

On the evening of his admission to the hospital he showed the following symptoms: Burning fever; skin dry and hot; tongue thickly coated, dry, red; intense thirst. Pulse small, tense, 110. Countenance expressive of depression of spirits; prostration of strength; lies in any position; no headache; slightly flighty.

Marked dyspnœa; respiratory movements frequent and small.

The cough is frequent and distressing, with a sensation of constriction along the base of the thorax, as if it were laced with a band of iron. He raises a little gummy sputa which strongly adheres to the bottom of the vessel.

Percussion yields a good sound every where, except at the posterior and inferior portion of the right side, where the dulness is, however, very faint. But in this region a loud bellows'-murmur is heard, without crepitation or mucous rattle, and a diffuse bronchophony extending to the axilla.—Water and sugar; *Aconite* and *Bryonia* 18, in alternation.

March 23.—Fever the same, pulse more frequent, 120. Increased prostration; anxiety. A little flighty.

Oppression, respiration rapid and small.

Cough less frequent, but distressing, and followed by expectoration of viscid, gummy sputa, not very abundant.

The dulness behind is more distinct; bronchial murmur very harsh, and mingled with a few isolated vesicles of mucous rattle. The murmur has spread over a larger surface, as far as the spine of the shoulder-blade; the bronchophony likewise.—*Bryonia*, two solutions.

In the evening, the oppression is much worse, the cough and expectoration become much less. Delirium.

March 24.—Skin dry, burning; tongue thickly coated, red, covered in the middle with a little brownish and dried-up mucus. Pulse small, filiform, hurried. Countenance sinking; look staring, extinct. Delirium. The patient is unable to sit up in bed without support.

Breathing irregular, unequal.

No cough, no expectoration.—*Belladonna*, in solution; a solution of twenty-five centigrammes of tartar-emetic. Blister.

No auscultation was employed, because the patient was too weak.

March 25.—Same as yesterday. Auscultation reveals mucous rattle, with large vesicles behind and in front below the right nipple. On the left side, under the clavicle, bronchial murmur is heard.—Tartar-emetic, in solution, two blisters.

March 26.—Pulse still smaller, filiform, hurried. Fuligo on the lips and gums. Twice last night the patient was comatose.

Breathing intermittent; tracheal rattle.

Mucous rattle in the right side of the thorax, very distinct below the nipple; bronchial murmur, mingled with mucous rattle under the left clavicle.—Tartar-emetic.

March 27.—Tracheal rattle, coldness and blueness of the extremities. Face covered with a clammy sweat.—March 28th, death.

Post-mortem examination, 36 hours after his death: 1st, white hepatization of the whole right lung, with a small quantity of purulent effusion in the corresponding pleural cavity and false membranes, which cause strong adhesions between the posterior portion of the lower lobe and the pleura costalis. 2d, similar hepatization of the upper portion of the left lung in a space of four fingers'-breadth; the remaining portion of the lungs is only congested, of a dark color, similar to that of a sediment of claret wine. No alterations in the pleura. The arachnoïd, and the pia-mater of the two anterior lobes of the brain on a level with the frontal eminences, are of a uniform, bright-red color, which does not disappear by washing, in an extent of about two centimeters on the right, and about three on the left side. Along the boundaries of this congestion, these same membranes present an arborescent appearance of injected vessels, which gradually becomes less and less, until it disappears in the healthy tissue. The subjacent cerebral tissue in the centre of these lesions is injected and softened at the surface. Otherwise there is no effusion either of serum or pus in these parts, nor is there any where else in the cavity of the skull.

When I saw this patient for the first time, on the morning of the seventh day of the sickness, I looked upon the suppuration as imminent, or perhaps as having already set in, and I deemed the patient's life as good as lost.

On the night before he died, he had been prescribed a solution of *Aconite*, and one of *Bryonia*, which he took alternately. The Bryonia was continued for thirty-six hours longer. Its inefficacity having become apparent, we had recourse to *Tartarus-emeticus*, and applied a large blister on the right side. This treatment was likewise without any avail, and the patient died on the twelfth day.

In my opinion this patient would have died under any treatment. To judge from previous cases, where Bryonia had had a good effect in spite of the advanced stage and the intensity of the disease, it seemed to me that this remedy might likewise prove useful in the present case. Owing to the fact that this drug frequently occasions a momentary aggravation, which is succeeded by a remission of the symptoms, the medicine was continued next day. Instead of a remission, the disease continued to progress towards a fatal termination. Tartar-emetic and blisters were resorted to on the same evening. I discontinued the strictly Hahnemannian treatment because its continuation in the present case would have seemed to me no better than *pure empiricism*, which I do not approve of. Will it be objected that a continuation of the homœopathic treatment would have rendered its want of success still more striking? This want of success seemed to me to have been sufficiently manifest to authorize me to discontinue the treatment.

I have asked myself: Could this patient have been cured under any kind of treatment?

Let me remind the reader of Roman's antecedents, his privations, his misery, his grief, his progressive debility, until the moment when he was taken sick, of the absence of all care and treatment until the sixth day of his pneumonia, and lastly, of the intensity of his disease at the time when he arrived at the hospital, and the termination in suppuration both in the right and left lung will not seem surprising.

I should like to be told what treatment will, in a similar case, result in a cure without fail. I confess I am ignorant of any such treatment. I am willing to admit, however, that, when I saw the patient for the first time, the suppurative process may not yet have commenced. I might be told that I have reported cases of other patients who remained eight or nine days without any treatment, and who got well nevertheless. This is true; but not one of these patients, on their admission to the hospital, was as low as Roman, nor had they been exposed to influences that were as favorable to suppuration as was the case in the present instance.

Considering all things I am disposed to believe that the homœopathic method failed in the present case. When the tartar emetic was resorted to, the patient was past all chances of recovery; this agent cannot, therefore, be held accountable for the failure.

CASE 40.—*Pneumonia of the left lung.*

On the 15th of July, 1848, the man Causse, nightman,

was admitted in the ward St. Benjamin, No. 2. He was 60 years old, of a strong constitution, and habitually in the enjoyment of good health. For the last eight days he had been sick. From the commencement of his sickness he had had a violent fever with cough, bloody sputa, and a painful stitch under the axilla. Not considering himself very sick, he had not sent for any physician, and had simply dieted himself, had kept his bed, and had only commenced last night to take some gum-water, on account of feeling worse than usual. This is all we could gather from the incoherent and incomplete answers that this patient returned to our questions an hour after his admission.

He was very weak. Face pale, forehead covered with a clammy sweat; tongue dry, with a blackish coating, fuligo on the lips and teeth; skin dry and burning; pulse quick and small. Breathing embarassed; distressing sense of oppression, especially in the left chest.

Cough not frequent, difficult; sputa scattering, of the color of prune-juice. To examine the patient, he has to be supported while sitting up in bed, after which he falls back like a dead mass. Percussion yields a perfect dulness of sound in the posterior and inferior two-thirds of the left thorax. Auscultation reveals a bellows'-murmur in the same region, intermingled with large and humid mucous rattle, especially at the base, and bronchophony. —Water and sugar; *Bryonia* 12, and *Carbo-veget.* 12, in solution, alternately. Large blister behind, in the region of the lungs.

About 10 o'clock at night, the oppression became worse; the hands were cold and the nails blue; face hippocratic, with cold sweat on the forehead and temples. On the rest of the body the skin was dry and hot; pulse small and very rapid.

Cough rare; no expectoration; delirium, and next morning, death.

Post-mortem examination 36 hours after death: Puru lent effusion of about a quarter of a pound in weight in the left pleural cavity. The lower lobe of the left lung was found covered with false membranes, and the whole parenchyma was infiltrated with pus.

CASE 41.—*Pneumonia of the right lung.*

The widow Letandin, 58 years old, a fleshy and robust woman, was admitted in the ward Sainte-Anne No. 17, on the 8th of September, 1848.

She was delirious, and no information could be obtained from her concerning her previous state. A patient who knew her, told us that she was addicted to drinking, and that she had been in good health on the 29th of August last.

The following were her symptoms: Countenance sunken; icteric color of the skin, with pungent heat; anxiety, restlessness, and plaintive cries.

Pulse small, 120. Tongue dry and covered in the middle with a brownish coating, intense thirst. The patient begs for drink all the time.

Excessive oppression; short and hurried breathing; the patient who is scarcely able to articulate, complains of a dull pain in the right breast.

Coughs but seldom, without raising any thing.

Dulness under the right clavicle, and on a level with the supra- and sub-spinal depressions.

Bronchial respiration in the same region, with large and humid crepitation in front, and behind only in the supra-spinal depression.—*Bryonia* 12, in solution.

Sept. 9.—Constant restlessness and delirium during the night.

In the morning the face was yellow and blueish, the sclerotica and the skin of the body yellow.

Pulse smaller and more hurried.

Breathing short, with cold breath.

No cough, nor any expectoration.—*Bryonia* and *Iodine* 3, in alternation.

In the evening the patient tried to get up several times. The restlessness continued to increase; coma set in in the night. The eyes are sunken and wandering, the hands and lips blue and cold; colliquative diarrhœa. —Death.

Post-mortem ex.:—Purulent infiltration of the superior lobe of the right lung. At the base of this lobe a thin layer of red hepatization is seen; the middle lobe is similarly hepatized; the lower lobe is congested.

I have related these two cases, in order to substantiate my previous assertion: that two patients who died in my wards, could not properly be counted in the number of my cases. I do not think that any treatment ought to be expected to raise the dead.

REFLECTIONS.

I have thus related forty cases of pneumonia. It might be observed, perhaps, that I ought to have related all the cases which I have treated, in order to furnish a complete statistical series. I have not adopted this method for the simple reason that I have not yet felt authorized to place the old-school treatment of pneumonia in such an evident position of inferiority, as it would undoubtedly have occupied, if I had related every case. For it would have been found that all the patients who came to my wards before suppuration had set in, were cured except one. Even if I had not directed particular attention to this fact, others would have done it for me, and the result would have been the same. I have been desirous of avoiding a premature conclusion, and collecting a great number of data before pronouncing my final verdict.

I shall not yet compare the result of Hahnemann's method with those of other methods of cure. I shall do this at a later period after having accumulated all the facts upon which such a comparison should be based. Even if I had intended to institute such a comparison, the data for it do not exist. Most of our statistical tables are intended to demonstrate the superiority either of blood-letting, or tartar-emetic, or blisters. Every author simply wished to express his predilections or antipathies in numbers.

To compare the two methods satisfactorily, each ought to be employed with all its means and resources and all its conditions of success. Where do we find a statistical table of pulmonary inflammations treated in this manner? Those who treat them well, do not count them.

I shall content myself with calling the attention of the reader to one point. Might not the cure of my cases be attributed to a natural tendency inherent in pneumonia to get well, provided the course of the disease were not interfered with?

At first sight, this objection seems specious. It is the last refuge of the opposition, and it is incumbent upon the opponents to prove the truth of our denial. I ask, therefore, upon what grounds could one claim such constant and brilliant success for the expectant method, in other words, attribute them to a complete absence of all treatment, except a few very simple hygienic conditions?

Upon the ground of tradition? But the experience of the past is uniformly in favor of energetic treatment in pneumonia, if we wish to avoid fatal terminations. No sane man will deny that a pneumonia will sometimes get well of itself. But this is only an exception which confirms the rule.

Upon the ground of experience? The expectant method has not as yet, to my knowledge, any experience in its favor in regard to the treatment of pneumonia. I have seen some cases where pneumonia was systematically treated by mild means, such as purgatives, gentle blisters &c.; and I have been present at the post-mortem examinations of a few patients thus treated. I have seen patients who objected to any active treatment; these patients died almost without an exception, whenever the disease was well defined both locally and constitutionally. Who does not know these facts?

Upon the nature of the disease? But all authors consider pneumonia as a parenchymatous inflammation, which, if left to itself, and frequently in spite of all the efforts of art, terminates in suppuration or white hepatization. Is the termination in suppuration a fiction? Is the termination in induration a rare occurrence in our dissection-rooms? Are the clinical cases of Lænnec, Andral, Louis, Chomel, lists of mortality that were drawn up on purpose to frighten patients and physicians?

Upon the treatment? There is no more energetic treatment than that which is generally pursued in pneumonia; venesection after venesection, massive doses of tartar-emetic, blister after blister. It cannot be said that such a treatment simply aids the efforts of nature. We should have to explain in the first place in what way these repeated bleedings and the tartar-emetic aid nature, and which of these healing agents acts upon such vast functional derangements.

The objections drawn from the expectant method are unworthy of the scientific physician. Is it not evident that such objections fall with a crushing weight upon all the various modes of active treatment that have been pursued in pneumonia? What! you pretend to say that pneumonia is curable with pure water, and yet you treat this disease with bleeding after bleeding, with massive doses of tartar-emetic which are repeated day after day, and with blisters which render it impossible for the poor patient to lie on his bed without pain, and which cause sores, that cannot be dressed, without inflicting suffering? Is not this species of medicine, this kind of healing art the most cruel deception? These inferences necessarily follow from your assertions that my cases got well without any treatment.

What do the facts which I have related, show?

1. In all my patients the disease got worse until the treatment commenced.

2. Immediately after the treatment had been commenced, an aggravation that was previously expected, set in for about 24 hours, after which the symptoms decreased either partially or in their totality. From this moment the disease hastened towards a favorable termination. In some cases the improvement commenced without any previous aggravation, and continued without interruption.

3. Bryonia caused a remarkable decrease of the number of pulsations, from 20 to 30 in one day; and at the period when resolution commenced, the pulse came down from 110 or 120 to 60, 56 and even 44. In one case which I have not related, it fell to 36. I have seen it come down from 120 to 80 between the morning- and evening-visit, and from 120 to 60 between the two morning-visits.

4. In old persons who had been a whole week without any treatment, and in whom the termination in induration (chronic pneumonia) seemed inevitable, this termination did not take place in a single case. Only the physical signs of hepatization did not scatter as rapidly as in the other cases.

5. Suppuration did not set in in a single case where it did not already exist at the commencement of the treatment. In some cases it seems to have been arrested by the treatment; only in a single case it was either not prevented or not arrested; (the two patients who were brought to the hospital dying, cannot be counted, in my judgment.)

I am willing to make every possible allowance for crises and critical days; I do not say that the homœopathic treatment has such a perfect control over the disease, that its stages cease to be distinctly observable. But I know very well that, at the critical period, the crisis may be incomplete or false; I know that suppuration is also a crisis, and that it terminates fatally. I admit therefore that the homœopathic treatment does not remove the crises, but it substitutes successful and complete crises for false and incomplete ones.

If critical periods happened in most of the cases which I have related, we must not forget that the crisis which determines the final result, generally takes place nearest to the period when the treatment was commenced. This truth is another confirmation of the efficacy of the treatment which we have pursued.

CONCLUSION.

The Hahnemannian treatment of pneumonia seems to exercise a most happy influence over the symptoms, course and duration of this disease.

Hence I affirm that this mode of treatment should be made a subject of scientific analysis and observation.

www.ingramcontent.com/pod-product-compliance
Lightning Source LLC
LaVergne TN
LVHW021405110826
845150LV00007B/1796

* 9 7 8 1 4 2 5 5 1 2 1 7 0 *